Eczema! Cure It!

E
Cure It!

Find your food reactions

Experience perfect skin

Eliminate your triggers

Dr Rodney Ford
MD MBBS FRACP

Could you be reacting to foods?
Could you have *The Gluten Syndrome*?
Could your child have perfect skin?

This book can help you to systematically cure eczema.
Investigate the triggers of your child's eczema.

One-in-five people are affected by eczema.
Eczema can seriously affect your health.
Now you can do something about it!

Eczema!
Cure It!

Dr Rodney Ford
Copyright 2008

National Library of New Zealand Cataloguing-in-Publication Data
  Ford, Rodney, ‡d 1949-
  Eczema! Cure it! : find your food reactions, experience perfect skin, eliminate your triggers / Rodney Ford.
  Includes bibliographical references.
  ISBN 978-0-473-10773-4
  1. Eczema in children—Prevention. 2. Food allergy in children.
  I. Title.
  618.925105—dc 22

Published by RRS Global Ltd.
PO Box 25-360, Christchurch, New Zealand.
www.rodneyford.co.nz
Printed by Tien Wah Press, Singapore
2008

All rights reserved.
Without limiting the rights under the copyright reserved above, no part of this publication may be reproduced, stored in or introduced into a retrieval system, or transmitted, in any form or by any means (electronic, mechanical, photocopying, recording or otherwise), without the prior written permission of the copyright owner and the publisher of this book.

Jacket cover, art work and illustrations
by Liz Fazakarley of *Ford Design*.

Dedication

To my patients who have
made this book possible.

"Where observation is concerned,
chance favours only the prepared mind."

Louis Pasteur, 1854

Other books by Dr Rodney Ford

- The Energy Effect. Your questions answered
- Are You Gluten-Sensitive? Your questions answered
- The book for the Sick, Tired and Grumpy
- Full Of It! The shocking truth about gluten
- Going Gluten-Free. How to get started
- The Gluten-Free Lunch Book
- Gluten-Free Parties and Picnics
- The Gluten Syndrome: is wheat causing you harm?

About the author

Dr Rodney Ford
Professor
MB BS MD FRACP MCCCH ASM

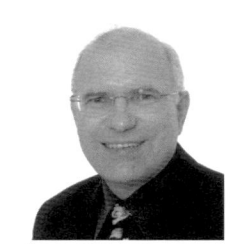

Dr Rodney Ford is a paediatric gastroenterologist, allergist and nutrition consultant. He is a former Associate Professor of Paediatrics at the Christchurch School of Medicine, University of Otago, New Zealand, and is recognized worldwide as an expert on adverse food reactions.

His major area of interest is the relationship between your food and your health – good or bad. In his clinics he is constantly seeing people who are suffering from eating foods that are making them ill. He has been interested in the relationship between eczema and food allergy for a long time. More recently he has discovered that gluten plays a large part in the pathophysiology of eczema.

Dr Ford graduated with Honours from the University of New South Wales in 1974 (MB BS). He went on to study food allergy and intolerance problems in New Zealand, Australia and the United Kingdom, was admitted as a Fellow of the Royal Australasian College of Physicians in Paediatrics (FRACP) in 1981 and was awarded his Doctorate of Medicine (MD) by the University of New South Wales in 1982 for his thesis titled *Food hypersensitivity in children: diagnostic approaches to milk and egg hypersensitivity*. This was regarded as a major work regarding the diagnosis of food allergies in children.

Dr Ford currently runs the *Children's Gastroenterology and Allergy Clinic,* a busy private clinic in Christchurch, New Zealand. He has written over one hundred scientific papers, including book chapters and entire books.

Contents

Introduction. Yes! It can be cured! 7
   Are there any secrets? 8

1. Why the controversy? 9
   Food allergy goes undiagnosed 10
   Cure it or cover it? 14

2. Eczema! What is it? 15
   What is eczema? 16
   The eczema progression 17
   What is the risk of getting eczema? 20
   Other types of eczema 21
   The eczema environment 22

3. Foods are the culprits! 23
   Foods in the womb 24
   How do foods cause eczema? 27
   Food chemical reactions 29

4. Eczema! Find your triggers! 31
   Skin-prick tests 32
   What allergens can be tested? 36
   Skin-prick tests are not the whole answer 40

5. Milk, egg and peanut! 41
   Cow's milk 41
   Eggs 47
   Peanuts 51
   Gluten 52

6. The Gluten Syndrome! 53
  Blair's long-awaited recovery 54
  Gluten known to cause skin disease 59
  Eczema blood tests 61
  More about gliadin 63
  Gluten eczema stories 64
  Think about the gluten-eczema link 66

7. Eczema! Switch it off! 67
  Good gut bugs 67
  The "allergy switch" theory 68
  Probiotics can stop eczema 69
  Probiotics can prevent eczema 70
  How do probiotics work? 71

8. Creams and potions! 73
  Moisturizers and oils 73
  Steroids 74
  Non-steroid anti-inflammatory creams 77

9. Eczema! Prevent it! 79
  Ten steps to prevent eczema 80
  1 - Before pregnancy: diet 80
  2 - During pregnancy: diet 81
  3 - Birth: probiotics 82
  4 - Infant feeding: breast feeding 83
  5 - Food skin-prick test: early identification 84
  6 - What formula? 85
  7 - Foods: cow's milk, eggs, peanuts, fish, gluten 86
  8 - Avoid inhalant allergens: house dust mite 87
  9 - Antihistamines: cetirizine 87
  10 - Supplements and skin care 89

References 91

Introduction. *Yes! It can be cured!*

Yes! Eczema can be cured! This is my experience from helping thousands of eczema-ridden children in my clinic. For most, their eczema can be cured.

I am a Paediatric gastroenterologist and allergist. Some people call me a "food doctor" because I help people find out what foods they should be avoiding, and what foods they should be eating. Most of the children I see have previously seen lots of doctors, including skin specialists, who usually prescribe yet more steroid creams.

A sense of frustration is often expressed by the parents of these children. They come to see me because the "standard medical approach" of yet more creams is not working. They want to avoid using these steroids if they can. They want an answer. Laila's story is typical:

Laila was five months old when I first saw her. Her parents told me that they had recently seen four general practitioners to help with her severe eczema. The first three doctors all prescribed various creams. But she did not get better. The fourth doctor suggested that Laila could be allergic to milk. So her mother who was still breastfeeding went dairy free, but with no benefit.

A few weeks later Laila was referred to me, she still had nasty eczema. Her skin-prick tests (an allergy test) showed that she had a severe reaction to egg. Her mother immediately removed all egg products from her diet and within a few weeks Laila got better. She also started to take a probiotic.

After two months her skin was almost perfect and she had no more need for steroid creams.

Are there any "secrets"?

Parents want a cure for their child's eczema! For most, I can help them get their skin back to almost perfect. However, there are no secrets! All the information offered in this book is from well-researched approaches to allergy and eczema. Sadly, these strategies only appear to be "secrets" because few people are aware of them.

Eczema can be cured!

The strategies I use to sort out the eczema puzzle are:
- Listen to the whole eczema story and work out any triggers;
- Do skin-prick-testing to discover foods or allergenic culprits;
- Order blood tests for allergy and immune function;
- Get blood tests done for gluten sensitivity;
- Work out an appropriate, low food-allergen diet;
- Deal with dust mites;
- Start probiotic treatment;
- Look at antihistamines to prevent asthma;
- Encourage the use of moisturisers;
- Use steroid creams sparingly;
- Prevent eczema and asthma for future children.

Currently, many medical doctors are unaware that eczema is commonly triggered by food allergy, so I have written this book to help children like Laila. My hope is that I can help many thousands of parents to overcome their frustrations with eczema. Eczema is a huge problem and it usually has a simple solution. This book presents you with the evidence and a plan of action. But first I would like to discuss some of the reasons for the controversy.

1. Why the controversy?

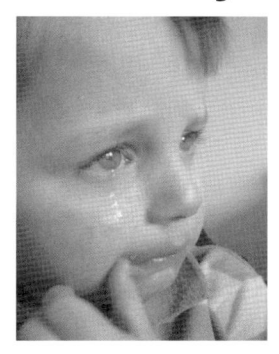

The idea that foods can cause eczema is controversial. But why is that so? There is a vast and convincing body of medical literature about food allergy. Food allergy has been researched for more than 50 years, so why is it still being ignored? I think that this divergence of opinion is more about "beliefs" than a genuine critique of the allergy data.

Most dermatologists remain unconvinced about food allergy causing eczema. Consequently, they continue to teach the "standard medical teaching" to the fledgling general practitioners: that eczema is merely a condition that allergy sufferers get, and that the treatment is skin care only (moisturizers and steroid creams).

Medics are skeptical about food allergy

As I have been studying food allergy for the last thirty years, I am surprised that so many of my medal colleagues remain skeptical about food allergy. A sense of frustration sometimes comes over me.

Food allergy goes undiagnosed

Every day I see children in my clinic with stories of suffering from eczema, sometimes for years. I recognise that they have a food allergy but this has gone undiagnosed. Their doctors had never even considered food allergy to be a possibility. Why isn't the allergy message getting through? Why are so many people suffering needlessly?

Sam, who is 15 months old and has severe eczema, came to see me with his mother. She said:

> "I have been to several dermatologists. I have tried all sorts of creams. But nothing seems to cure it. No one has ever suggested a food allergy. But I am suspicious about foods – I wonder if he is reacting to something he is eating. I am just not sure. I wonder if you can help me?"

There are a number of reasons for the poor uptake of the food allergy message.

Fringe element

Food allergy is thought by some people to be fad or a fringe diagnosis. However, the medical literature shows that 5-10% of children suffer from some sort of food allergy reactions. That means that up to one child in ten is affected; this is a sizable and common medical problem. Their symptoms such as eczema, runny noses, cough, gastric reflux, diarrhoea and constipation are treated as something to be masked. They are not recognised in the context of possible food allergy. The complete allergy picture is not seen.

Mum asks "please can you help me?"

Drugs not diet policy
The medical fraternity has been conditioned by the pharmaceutical industry to treat symptoms with medications and creams. Few pharmaceutical companies advocate dietary treatments. It would not be in their best interests to do so.

The standard skin specialist approach is to use stronger steroid creams for longer periods. Short appointment times help to promote this model of treatment. It is more efficient in the clinic to prescribe medication rather than spend the extra time sorting out the food triggers and subsequently manage a complex condition of multiple food allergies.

Lack of experience about allergy
I attend allergy and gastroenterology medical conferences. The other delegates are similar to me: allergy specialists who want to learn more and exchange information. However, general practitioners seldom turn up to these meetings. Also, food allergy is seldom part of a program drawn up for general practitioners. With little knowledge of food allergy, it is more comfortable to prescribe creams and quietly ignore the allergy issues.

Children are not just small adults
Dermatologists predominantly look after adults; their training is in the adult field. Under these circumstances, children are usually considered as if they are just small adults. But this is not the case. Babies and children have a different spectrum of allergic reactions that are not seen in adults as often. Also, skin prick testing is much more accurate in children than in adults. By contrast, adult food allergy is less common and skin prick tests are less reliable. You can see that it is easy for an "adult" dermatologist to infer from their adult experience that food allergy must be uncommon in *everyone*.

For example, an extract from a patient-information-sheet,(see www.skincarephysicians.com/eczemanet/index.html) published by the American Academy of Dermatology states: "There is no evidence that any dietary changes can help eczema sufferers. Some people believe that the exclusion of egg or cow's milk from children's diet may help, but exclusion diets can lead to a calcium or protein deficiency and may cause more harm than good."

They go on to say in their pamphlet: "Using too much steroid cream can cause thinning of the skin, making it more fragile and leading to blemishes, wrinkles or visible small blood vessels. Mild steroid creams, such as 1% hydrocortisone, are available over the counter from the chemist, but stronger ones need a prescription from a doctor."

This is what one of my mums (mother of Holly, 3 years old) said. She was irritated about advice given by her dermatologist:

> "I still feel cross! When Holly was about a year old, we took her to a skin specialist. She had bad eczema. We were told that there was only a very small percentage of children who had food-related eczema. We were also told that it was too hard to find out which foods could be possibly causing her the problem. This specialist also told us that the skin tests were very painful. But after seeing you, we at last know that Holly, now three years old, is food intolerant and that her eczema is definitely related to food".

> "I still feel very angry that we are now two years down the track without dealing with the food problems. Yes, it has taken us another two years to get to the stage where we could find out that food intolerance is a big factor for Holly and her eczema. It has been so frustrating."

> "By the way, another thing, the skin tests were fine, no trouble, no pain."

Another child, Anton, at six months of age, who was still on the breast, was seen by two specialists within a short space of time. I was subsequently asked to see him for his severe eczema and food allergies. Later, another paediatrician wrote to me saying:

> "Anton's mother does not need to continue her dairy-free diet ... as in most cases; the eczema is independent of major dietary factors."

Fortunately his mother did not heed this inaccurate advice. A few weeks later Anton was seen by a senior dermatologist who wrote this about Anton:

> "In the vast majority of children with atopic dermatitis, diet does not seem to be a significant factor. However, in Anton's case, there is certainly a suggestion that dairy allergy may be contributing, as he has improved since his mother has avoided dairy products – and he is virtually fully breast fed".

In this case, the dermatologist did acknowledge (although unusual) that dairy was the driving force behind Anton's eczema.

Parents often notice that food causes eczema

Cure it or cover it?

As you are aware, the customary medical strategy for treating eczema is to cover it with creams (Chapter 6 gives you the details). Moisturising creams help retain the water in the skin. Hydrocortisone creams and ointments certainly help to reduce the inflammation. Obviously, stronger steroids will suppress the inflammation even more successfully.

But steroid creams can be harmful in the long run. Long term use makes skin become thin and fragile. Capillaries will begin to show through. The pigmentation of skin can also be altered. A new type of non-steroid anti-inflammatory cream has been available for a few years. Two of these are "pimecrolimus" (trade name, Elidel) and tacrolimus (trade name, Protopic Ointment). They act to reduce the skin inflammation without the skin-thinning effect. However, these medications also need to be used with caution.

Unfortunately, none of these preparations will solve the underlying problem. These creams can only reduce and alleviate the symptoms. They definitely serve an important function in getting the eczema under control, but they are still a cover-up of the driving force behind most eczema.

My data shows that most people with eczema can be cured. In my clinical practice I have found that about 80% of children's eczema is driven by allergic food reactions. My goal is to have people get completely better, have perfect skin, and have no ongoing need for creams. The next chapter describes the eczema problem in more detail. Then we will look at how you can get better.

Eczema is more than skin deep

2. Eczema! What is it?

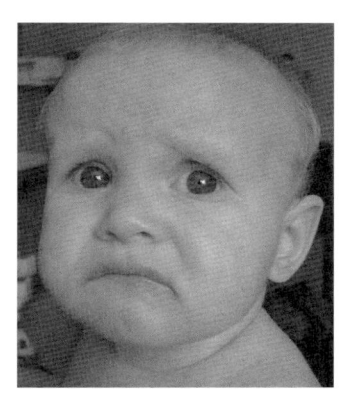

Why has your child got eczema? It's not fair! No one wants to have eczema. No one wants to have dry, rough, itchy skin. No one wants their face blemished by scars. No one wants to spend half the night scratching. What can you do about it?

My goal is a cure. I expect these children to have almost perfect skin within a few months of being on an appropriate diet along with applying a few other strategies and treatments to sort out their allergies. A food allergy is a contributing factor in about eight out of ten of these children. This is good news because if you can identify the offending allergy triggers, then the eczema can usually be cured.

I expect these children to be able to throw away most of their creams and potions. They will continue to have sensitive skin for a few more years and their skin may still feel a bit dry. However, a cure does not happen every time. Not everyone will respond, but that is my goal.

Strive for perfect skin

What is eczema?

Does your child really have eczema? Eczema is when you have patches of skin that are dry, red, scaly and itchy. It is an inflammation of the skin. In children it is also given the name "atopic dermatitis" – which means the eczema is associated with some sort of allergy. Sometimes it is called "baby eczema", or "infantile eczema". Medical research shows that eczema in children is often caused by some sort of allergic reaction.

> Most infant eczema is related to allergy

How does eczema feel?

A mum told me that they have given their son a nickname, "itchy-scratchy". That was because he was scratching all of the time, day and night as soon as he had a chance to get to his skin. This is one of the most typical things about eczema – the dreadful itchiness. Eczema is also called "the itch that rashes" or the itch that scratches". This is because the itchy skin (which can look quite normal and healed), when scratched, quickly produces the appearance of the typical eczema rash. If the skin is not scratched, then it looks healthy (but it can still be very itchy).

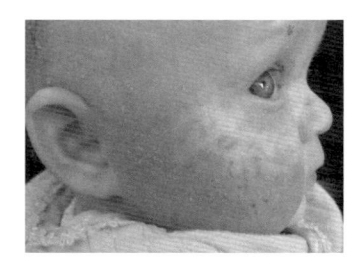

The eczema progression

Eczema can have a slightly different look from one person to the next . Eczema severity can also vary a great deal: it can be a mild, dry irritation, in small patches; it can be severe, with every part of the skin affected with cracked, weepy and sometimes infected skin; and it can be anything in between these extremes. Eczema also changes its appearance with age.

Babies

In babies, the eczema usually starts out as dry skin, little cracks behind the ears and a rough dry face in the first six weeks of life. Cracks and irritations often will occur on the cheeks. This is often associated with "cradle cap". (Cradle cap is a greasy, thick, yellowish, scaly rash associated with a type of fungal infection of the scalp – it is also called seborrhoeic dermatitis).

The cheeks can be bright red and the skin can be rubbed raw. After a few months, the eczema rash might progress to the chest, then to the back and then to the inside creases of the arms and legs. During this time, the skin can be infected, which gives it a weepy, crusty look. As the child learns to scratch, the skin will get damaged and deteriorate even more.

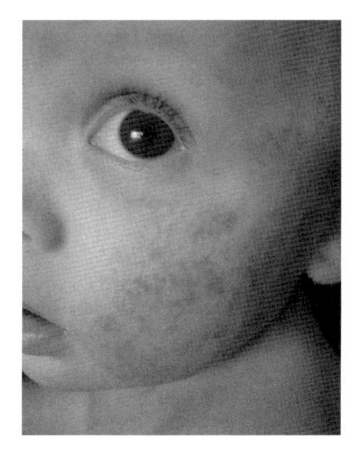

It is the scratching and the rubbing that damages the skin. The skin is so itchy that the child is driven to scratch and rip the skin. The skin will bleed and can easily get infected. If the skin gets a chance to heal, the skin will grow rough and thickened. Then this thick skin can easily crack, which hurts and stings. Often children will wake in the night scratching and crying out because they are so uncomfortable.

Toddlers
As the years go by, the pattern of eczema slowly changes. I think that this is because of the changing types of allergens that affect the skin. With age, the food allergies tend to be less of a problem, but then dust mite and gluten begin to trigger eczema. Often the face begins to settle down. The cheeks soften, but the creases of the arms and legs might get steadily worse.

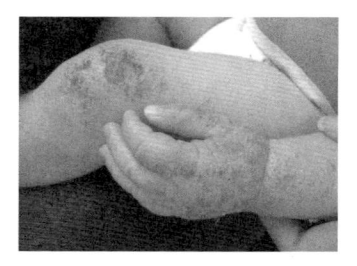

Eczema patterns change with age

What is it?

School age

Most eczema should have disappeared by school age. By five or six years old, the egg and cow's milk allergy, the triggers to so much eczema, should have resolved. At this age often the eczema is now on the outside areas of the arms and legs. Often the body is also rough and itchy. The creases are less of a problem. I find that the dust mite and gluten are the main culprits now.

knee (front)

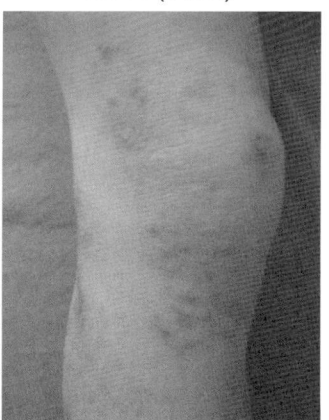

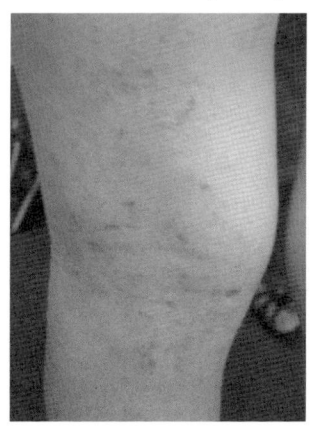

knee crease (back)

neck crease

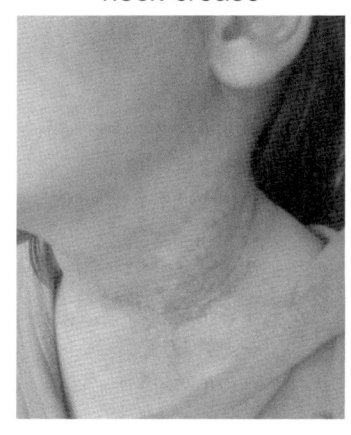

uncomfortable

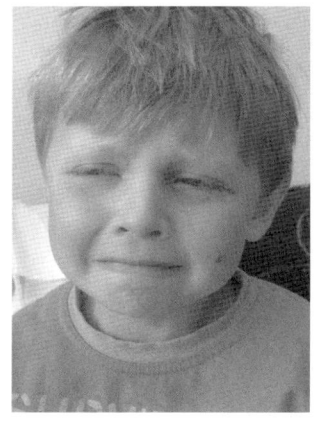

What is the risk of getting eczema?

Eczema is common. About a fifth (one in five, or 20%) of the population is affected in some way by eczema. Some of these children have very bad skin. The risk that you will get eczema is partly genetic:

o   If both of your parents have/had eczema, then your risk of getting eczema are about eighty percent (that is an 8 out of 10 chance).

o   If both of your parents have some sort of allergy (that is eczema, hay-fever or asthma), then your chance of developing eczema is about fifty percent (that is a 5 out of 10 chance).

o   If neither of your parents is affected by any allergies, then your chance of getting eczema is about ten percent (that is a 1 out of 10 chance).

From these figures you can see that your chance of getting eczema is related to your parents' allergic background. You can't change your parents! So instead, you have to deal with the eczema that you have and find a solution. That means paying close attention to your environment, your food, and your immunity.

One in five people get eczema

What is it?

Other types of eczema

Eczema is also known as "dermatitis" that means an inflammation of the skin. The focus of this book is on "atopic eczema/ dermatitis. However, there are other categories of eczema:

Allergic contact eczema: this is a red, itchy, weepy skin reaction. It occurs when the skin has come into contact with a substance that you are allergic to. Your immune system has recognized this substance as "foreign" and reacts against it. Things that can spark this sort of reaction include foods (especially egg white, peanut and cow's milk); poison ivy; and some preservatives found in creams and lotions.

Contact eczema: this is a localized reaction characterized by redness, itching, and burning. It occurs when your skin comes into contact with an irritant such as an acid, a cleaning agent, or other chemical.

Nummular eczema: these are coin-shaped patches of irritated skin. They are seen most commonly on the arms, the back, the buttocks, and then lower legs. These patches can be extremely itchy. They are persistent and hard to treat effectively.

Seborrhoeic eczema: these are yellowish, oily, scaly patches of skin. They are seen mostly on the scalp and the face.

Eczema shows up in various forms

The eczema environment

Although your genes are important, your environment plays a decisive role in the development of eczema. Eczema is due to a combination of your genes and your environment.

As you cannot change your genes, the only way to deal with your eczema is to change your environment and your own health. By understanding this, you might be able to cure your eczema. The environmental conditions that impact on your eczema include:

o   Early food exposure: pregnancy and breast feeding;
o   Introduction of milk and solids: the age started and the types of foods given;
o   The affect of gluten;
o   Birth bugs: the colonization of the colon with healthy bacteria;
o   Nutrition: the health of the skin is related to the quality of food that is consumed;
o   Skin care: how to cleanse and look after your skin.

These factors are discussed in detail in the next chapters.

3. Foods are the culprits!

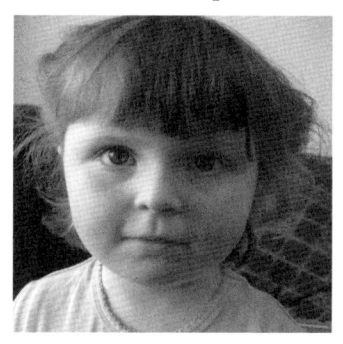

The first comprehensive study that proved that food can cause eczema was done by David Atherton, in London, in the 1970s. He studied 36 children who had eczema. It was a thorough study with a design called a "double-blind controlled crossover trial". The purpose was to see if a diet excluding dairy and egg products would influence their eczema: 20 children completed all parts of the study.

His results were startling: 14 children (70%) responded more favourably to the antigen-avoidance diet than to the control diet, whereas only one (5%) in the control diet group had a good response. Of interest, there was no correlation between a positive skin-prick test (SPT) to egg and cow milk antigen and response to the trial diet (see an explanation for this in the next chapter).

In a later study, Guillet (1992) assessed over 250 children with eczema. He noted that increased severity of eczema in the younger patients was directly correlated with the presence of food allergy.

Research proves foods can cause eczema

More recently, Werfel (2004) studied all of the allergy research that he could find and came to the conclusion: "Multiple clinical studies have addressed the role of food allergy in eczema. These show that elimination of relevant food allergens can lead to improvement in skin symptoms; that repeat challenge can lead to redevelopment of symptoms; and that the disease can be partially prevented by eliminating highly allergenic foods from the diets of infants and possibly breastfeeding mothers."

Clearly, there is much written in the medical literature to prove that foods can cause eczema. Let's look at the details.

Foods in the womb

Once a baby has been conceived and is growing in the mother's womb, the baby gets exposed to fragments of food from the mother's diet. The amniotic fluid (the watery liquid which surrounds the baby in the womb) contains these small amounts of food proteins that the mother has eaten. In the womb, the baby actually swallows this amniotic fluid.

Babies come into contact with foods in the womb

It is thought that this early exposure to the mother's foods helps guide the child in later life about what is safe to eat. Also this early exposure should help the baby develop a tolerance to these foods. Unfortunately, this can sometimes go wrong. In susceptible babies from allergic families, this very early food exposure (especially to egg) can develop into early allergic food reactions. Subsequently, it can lead to eczema.

Food proteins in breast milk
It is now widely recognized that breast milk is the very best milk to feed a baby. Breast milk is the perfect milk for your growing baby. Importantly, breast milk contains tiny amounts

of the foods that the mother eats. These food proteins help condition the baby to these tastes and flavours so that in the future, the introduction of foods will not be problematic. (Children are more likely to refuse foods that they haven't tasted through the mothers breast milk.)

Foods come through the breast milk

When food proteins are sought in breast milk, they can be found. Although the quantities of these foods are very small, they are clinically significant for the allergic child. Numerous medical studies show that babies can develop allergic symptoms from the food fragments of cow's milk, egg, and peanut coming through the mother's breast milk. Other foods, especially gluten, can also cause trouble.

Amelia is 12 months old. She had positive skin prick tests to milk, egg and wheat. Her mum said:

> "To begin with, Amelia had dreadful allergies. She had eczema all over her face, so it looked like she had slapped cheeks all the time. She was just miserable with trying to scratch. We brought her to see Dr Ford and she got skin-prick tested. We discovered that she was allergic to dairy, peanuts and eggs."
>
> "So, I started taking those foods out of her diet – well out of my diet mainly, because I was still breastfeeding her. Of course, I removed any traces of these foods from her diet as well – whatever she was eating. Because at that stage she wouldn't eat solids."
>
> "When I was still breastfeeding, her eczema improved – it began to clear up almost straight away. But the trouble was that her weight gain wasn't happening and

she wasn't eating any solids. Although I had taken these foods out of my diet, unfortunately, there must still have been traces of some trouble foods going through my breast milk."

"She didn't get fully better until she went onto the special low allergen milk (*Neocate*) – not long after that she started eating solids. As soon as she was on this strict diet, her growth came back up. And best of all, now her skin is beautifully clear and we don't have to use any creams on her at all. She is also gaining in weight! Fantastic!"

Colic and cow's milk
Relief from colic has been observed in breast fed infants whose mothers have been put onto a diet free of both cow's milk and dairy products. The baby's colic was found to return when the mother began eating dairy products again. These initial studies were done in 1978 by Jacobsson and Lindberg. These were "open" studies (mothers knew whether or not they were drinking cows' milk) which showed that a third of colicky babies responded to their mothers going off dairy.

This work was subsequently strongly criticized, and so they repeated their research by doing "double blind" studies (they gave the mothers "disguised" drinks so that they did not know which days they were drinking cows' milk). The mothers then observed the symptoms in their babies. By doing this more rigorous study, they confirmed their observations: that the colicky babies responded to dairy products. However, this time around they found that a quarter (25%: one in four) of colicky babies got better when their mother went on a dairy free diet.

Cow's milk can cause colic

How do foods cause eczema?

A wide number of foods can precipitate eczema. How does this happen? These foods can trigger eczema through a number of different mechanisms:
- by immediate allergic reactions;
- by slow onset (delayed) reactions;
- and by chemical irritation.

There are a number of different mechanisms that can set off eczema. Consequently, any single test is unlikely to identify all of the foods that could be contributing to the problem. Therefore, solving the eczema puzzle needs to take into account many factors including the history of the illness, the patterns of eczema, allergy tests, blood test results, and response to treatment.

The next step is to look at the types of food reaction in more detail.

Immediate allergic reactions
Immediate reactions to foods are the easiest to identify. The medical term for immediate reactions is "IgE-mediated reactions". This means that if a food is eaten, or even touches the skin, a reaction to that food will be seen within a few minutes. However, if tiny amounts of this food are given on a regular basis (usually this happens through the breast milk), then an immediate reaction to that food is difficult to pick up.

The baby will start to get frequent rashes and then eczema will start to develop, especially on the face and cheeks. Because only tiny amounts of protein from the mother's food are getting to the baby every day, the offending food may not be immediately obvious. However, these types of food allergy can be readily identified by skin-prick testing (see next chapter).

Slow-onset allergic reactions
Reactions to foods can also occur slowly. This means a reaction happens hours or even days after eating a food. These slow-onset adverse reactions are more difficult to identify. This is because there is not a close relationship between the time that the food is eaten and when the adverse reaction occurs. Also, under these slow-onset circumstances, skin prick tests are negative to the offending foods.

Skin-patch testing has recently been demonstrated as a useful technique to reveal these delayed onset foods reactions. To do a patch-test, a small amount of the food in question is put onto the skin and covered with a special adhesive patch. It is left in place for 24–48 hours. The patch is then removed and skin is examined to see if an allergic reaction has taken place. (This often provokes a patch of eczema at the test site.)

Food reactions can take days to show up

The most common foods to cause delayed onset reaction are gluten and dairy. Blood tests can be done to look at the IgG-antibody levels of these two foods. High antibody levels suggest that the body's immune system is reacting to these foods. In turn, that means it is worthwhile giving a trial of a gluten-free and/or dairy free-diet if indicated by these blood tests.

It is my experience that for babies (under twelve months of age) dairy is the most common slow-onset food reaction. When dairy is removed from their diet, often the eczema dramatically improves. For toddlers and older children, I have observed that gluten plays the most important role in their eczema (see Chapter 6).

Food chemical reactions

Every single thing that you put into your mouth is made up of chemicals. There are many thousands of different chemicals that get combined to make up the hundreds of varieties of foods that you eat. It is this vast assortment of chemicals that give your foods their characteristic colours, flavours and textures. Unfortunately, many of these natural food chemicals can also cause food reactions.

Non-allergic food intolerance

Yes, naturally occurring food chemicals can spark off skin reactions. Some of these food chemicals have the ability to trigger the release of "histamine" from the allergy cells (mast cells) in the skin. This is a chemical irritation, rather than an allergic reaction. This can lead to histamine flare-ups of eczema – especially around the mouth and cheeks.

Histamine is a substance that makes the skin very itchy. It is the substance that makes a mosquito bite itchy. The more the skin is scratched, the worse the eczema becomes.

This chemical histamine release is usually seen as an immediate flare reaction around the mouth (called: non-immunological contact urticaria) to benzoic acid from citrus fruits in children (this is especially seen in children with atopic eczema).

Other food additives and colourings can also have this effect. Additives such as sulphites, salicylates, tartrazine and monosodium glutamate (MSG) are implicated in these flare-up reactions of urticaria and eczema.

Chemicals can provoke eczema

Oral-Allergy-Syndrome

Perhaps the best known type of chemical food reaction is called the "oral-allergy-syndrome". This is a chemical reaction to foods which is felt in your mouth. It is found especially when the following foods are eaten fresh, raw and early in the season:

- Fruits: apple, peach, plum, nectarine, cherry.
- Vegetables: tomato, celery, carrot.
- Nuts: almond, hazel, walnut.

The oral allergy syndrome is characterized by a local itching or swelling in the lips, the mouth, the tongue and sometimes the throat. Some people experience a burning sensation. This happens almost immediately (within minutes) after coming in contact with the food. The good news is that these irksome food chemicals (found in these fruits and vegetables) can be destroyed by heating. Consequently, for the relief of most sufferers, when these foods are cooked, these chemicals no longer cause a reaction.

Some children, as well as having this oral-allergy-syndrome, will also break out in eczema when exposed to these natural food chemicals. Such flare-ups can occur within minutes. This subsequent scratching can quickly make a mess of their skin.

The birch pollen connection

The mechanism behind the oral-allergy-syndrome reaction can be due to cross-reactivity to other pollen allergens (especially from birch pollen), or to food chemicals causing a release of histamine in the mouth and creating exactly the same symptoms of an allergic reaction. Many other chemicals and irritants can cause eczema flare-ups when in direct contact with the skin: for instance washing powders, wool and fabrics can all cause such irritation. These aggravators need to be identified before the eczema skin can fully heal.

4. Eczema! Find your triggers!

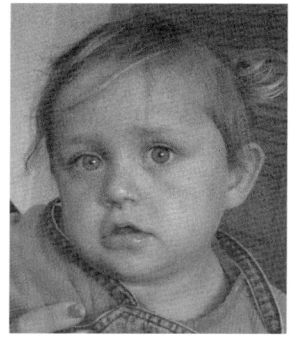

You cannot change your genetic make-up, but you *can* change your external environment. By "external environment" I mean everything that surrounds you. That is: all of the foods you eat; the pollens you are exposed to in the air (called aero allergens or inhalant allergens); the allergens in your bedding (especially the dust mites); and the hair and dander from your pets.

Your "internal environment" is also important to your wellbeing. By this I mean: your choices of food (some foods can make you sick); the state of your immune system (this needs attention in eczema as in other illness), and your mental attitude (your emotions directly affect your health).

The early foods cause the problem
The medical research mentioned in the previous chapter shows that food allergy contributes hugely to baby eczema. It turns out that the foods that we are exposed to early in life, and for the longest period of time, cause us the most problems. So, in most western countries, it is the dairy products, the soy and the eggs that cause most of our eczema problems.

Suspect early foods

By contrast, in Denmark for example, where there is a strong, continuing tradition of eating herring and cod, there is a higher incidence of herring and cod allergies in these children. Yet again, in Eastern countries, where sesame seeds are consumed in larger quantities, sesame seed allergy is a common problem. However, as we get older, foods play a lesser role in eczema reactions.

Food triggers?

So how do you find out what foods are causing the problem? What tests are available?

These allergic food reactions are mostly due to an allergic response to various food *proteins*. They are immune responses. The best way to detect *immediate* food allergy reactions is by skin prick tests.

Skin prick testing

Yes, it is my experience that skin-prick tests for foods are extremely useful. They are also safe, painless and simple to do. This is a precise way to identify the offending foods.

Skin-prick tests are gentle

Eczema cannot be properly managed without discovering the foods and inhalants that are the culprits setting off the eczema cycle. Skin prick testing identifies possible allergens. When done properly, it is a gentle test.

How is it done?

Skin-prick testing is simple and should be pain free. After marking the back (or forearm) with a pen, a small droplet of oil that contains the specific allergen (a food or an aero-allergen) is placed on the skin. This is usually done on the back, for babies and toddlers, and on the forearm for older children and adults.

pen mark

droplet of allergen

gentle prick

skin reaction

Next, the skin surface is very gently pricked through this droplet. It is a very superficial prick, a light touch on the skin. I use a 23 guage needle.

A positive test starts to occur within a few minutes. After 5–10 minutes a small wheal (like a little mosquito bite) develops. The size of the reaction (the wheal size) is measured at 10–15 minutes. It can get a little itchy but settles down in about half an hour.

In children, skin prick testing is accurate. With age, the skin-prick tests tell you more about past food allergies rather than present clinical intolerances. Therefore in adults, skin tests for foods are less useful.

How does it work?
The skin-prick test measures immediate reactions. It is a test that measures the "IgE-sensitivity" to the allergens which have been pricked gently into the skin. As soon as the allergen gets into the skin, it comes in contact with the allergy cells in your skin (the mast cells, which are packed full of histamine). If your mast cells have been sensitized to that allergen, they will immediately release their histamine, and this creates the wheal, just like a mosquito bite.

The skin-prick test is a biological reaction and takes about 10–15 minutes to get to its maximum intensity.

If the child has been treated with an antihistamine within the preceding 24 hours, then the skin tests will be attenuated. In other words reactions will be less dramatic and will take longer to show up.

Skin-prick tests accurately identify food allergens

Who should get tested?

I recommend that all babies, all children and all adults with eczema or asthma should be tested with a selection of skin-test allergens. All breastfed babies with eczema need skin-prick testing. All people who have troublesome allergy symptoms should be investigated by skin-prick tests. Consequently, in my clinic, I do skin-prick testing for all children with eczema.

Skin-prick tests can be done at any age: even on new-born babies (although it is less reliable at this age). It is my routine practice to do the first set of skin-prick tests at about three months of age. By this age the baby has developed the capacity to mount a specific IgE-response in the skin. But, if the baby has bad eczema in the first few weeks of life, then it is useful to do the skin tests earlier.

This is especially helpful in breastfed babies with eczema. Most of the time these babies are reacting to food proteins that are coming through in their mother's breast milk. By accurately identifying what the baby's skin is reacting to in the breast milk, I can then advise the mother about what foods that she should be avoiding in her diet. Usually, the eczema will completely go away. For instance, Thomas's mum said:

> "Knowing what foods to avoid, by the skin tests, made the world of difference. As soon as I cut eggs out of my diet (I was breastfeeding) his skin cleared up."

Detects problem food allergens in breast milk

What allergens can be tested?
There are two categories of allergens that you can be tested for: food and inhalants.

Foods: The most common and useful foods to test for are:
o	cow's milk
o	egg white
o	peanut
o	fish
o	tree nuts
o	wheat
o	soy

In adults, testing for shellfish is important. Usually, food reactions to fruits and vegetables cannot be successfully tested by skin tests – that is because these fruit and vegetables reactions are usually caused by the chemicals in these foods, rather than by the food proteins.

Inhalants: The important inhalant allergens (also called aero-allergens) are:
o	house dust mite
o	grass pollens (rye grass, timothy grass)
o	tree pollens (especially birch)
o	animal dander (cat fur, dog hair, horse hair, and feathers).

Who can do skin tests?
Most allergists do their own skin-prick testing. I carry out skin-tests on my patients as a routine part of their normal consultation. This gives me the opportunity to interpret their results as soon as they come up, and in context with their clinical story. They are also useful because they can give immediate answers to the eczema triggers.

Also, many medical laboratories are set up to perform skin-prick tests. You can ask your doctor to refer you to one of these laboratories for these tests. Yes, you should ask for skin-prick tests to help identify any suspected allergens if you have eczema, asthma, hay-fever and suspected food allergy. Many doctors do not understand the value of these skin-prick tests so they need to be encouraged to request these tests.

If you are not able to get these skin tests done, then another option is to get the IgE blood tests: these are called EAST (enzyme allergosorbent test) or RAST (radio allergosorbent test) tests. These tests give you the same information as the skin-tests. They test for levels of "specific IgE antibodies" in the blood to each of the allergens of interest.

When should skin tests be repeated?
It is good news that most food allergies go away as you get older. Coinciding with this, the skin-prick tests also wane with age. That means carrying out regular skin-prick testing is useful in tracking the current status of the food allergy. Also, repeating the skin-prick tests help to confirm to the parents that they are indeed making a difference by strictly controlling their child's diet.

It is my practice to conduct skin-prick tests at the ages of 3–6 months, 12 months, 2 years, 3 years, 5 years, 8 years and 12 years. I find that giving them accurate feed-back about the progress of their allergies is extremely helpful.

Repeat skin-prick tests every year or so

Monika's story:

A concerned mum, Monika, wrote to me about her baby boy. I am told similar stories most days. She says:

> "I would really appreciate your advice. My son is 6 months old, and has suffered from flare-ups of his eczema since very young (as well as cradle cap). He has been only had breast milk up to now. His eczema has moved from covering his back, to his tummy and now to his legs (it is worst behind his knees). It is now beginning on his face."

> "We have been very careful with any contact (no laundry liquid, all cotton clothing etc). I have tried a wide variety of emollients on him with no improvement, other than hydrating the skin for an hour or two! Reluctantly, I am now trying a steroid (hydrocortisone) cream. I have heard that 'allergy parents' may be the reason for infantile eczema."

> "I have mild asthma and hay-fever and my husband has a very small patch of eczema himself. Would this be why our son has eczema? Or could this be a food allergy coming through my breast milk?"

> "What action (blood tests/ skin-prick tests etc?) would you recommend? We can't just sit and watch his eczema get worse. Our doctors have just generalised the condition – hoping that he may just grow out of it. Many thanks in advance, Monika."

My reply was:
"Yes I can help. I suggest the following:
1) Get skin prick tests if you can – especially to egg, milk and peanut.

2) Start a probiotic.
3) Whilst breastfeeding you will probably need to go off dairy, egg and peanut.
4) Yes, use a 1% hydrocortisone cream for another month.
5) Avoid all egg, dairy and peanut in his solids.

I hope that this helps. With appropriate management I expect nearly all babies to get completely better."

Monika wrote back a few days later:

> "I'm so glad that you pointed me in the right direction. The doctors who I saw took a lot of convincing – or should I say begging – to get the skin pricks and bloods done. I could see my diet was already making a difference before the tests so I was convinced he was allergic to some of the foods that I had been eating."

A few weeks later she wrote again:

> "I am just following up on our earlier email exchange. Our baby son had the skin-prick tests and blood tests. This showed he had allergies to dairy and peanut. Since avoiding these foods in my diet, my breastfed son's eczema is 95% resolved. Just thought you'd like to hear that your advice was spot on. And the relief we feel is unexplainable! Many thanks. Best Regards, Monika."

This baby is typical. His eczema would have gotten progressively worse if mum had not changed her diet. The skin test helped mother work out what foods she needed to avoid. Because the skin tests gave her certainty about her diet, it was easier for her to comply.

Skin prick tests are not the whole answer

But skin tests are not the whole answer. This is because many foods, especially dairy and gluten can cause the delayed onset type of reaction. Under these circumstances, the skin tests are negative for dairy and gluten.

If the skin-prick tests are negative, then dairy or gluten should still be suspected. To make a diagnosis of gluten-sensitivity, blood tests are needed. Should the eczema not settle – again blood tests are needed to check out immune function.

Food reactions are not the only cause of eczema. Next, we will look at the main food culprits in more detail.

5. Milk, egg and peanut!

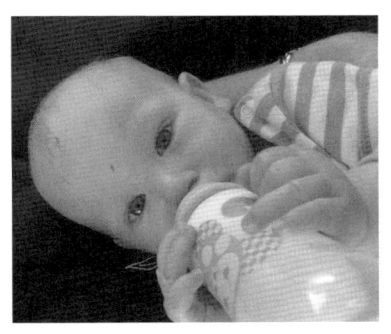

The most common culprits that precipitate eczema are the foods cow's milk, hen's eggs, peanuts, and gluten. We will look at each of these in detail.

As mentioned previously, the earlier a food is introduced, the more likely it is to cause an allergy. This is one of the reasons to advise later introduction of solids to children who have a family history of allergy. The advice is, if possible, to delay their first solids until over six months. Furthermore, avoid the strong food allergens (milk, egg, peanut, gluten soy and fish) until after 12 months old.

Cow's milk

It is said that cow's milk is produced for a baby cow – the calf, and human breast milk is produced for a baby human – the child. Cow's milk is so inappropriate for a baby to drink that it has to be extensively modified to make it safe for the baby to drink.

Avoid cow's milk if possible

Cow's milk is a common allergen

Cow's milk is a very common trigger for baby eczema. Cow's milk is one of the first food proteins to which most children are exposed, either in a formula or through the mother's breast milk. Children who are allergic to cow's milk will often be allergic to other foods, especially eggs and peanuts. For those children who are allergic to cow's milk, it is important to find them a safe alternative drink. There are a number of choices depending on the age of the child.

What is good about cow's milk?
Cow's milk has lots of goodness in it. Cow's milk has a number of components which include: the proteins (whey and casein), the sugar (lactose) and the fat. It also contains lots of minerals and vitamins. It is especially valued for its protein and its high concentration of calcium. However, cow's milk is not an essential food. All of its nutrients can be readily obtained from other foods. Cow's milk and its derivatives (cheese, yoghurt, butter) are convenient and taste good, although not necessary.

What is bad about cow's milk?
The lactose is not the problem. Cow's milk contains about 5% lactose, and human breast milk has about 7% lactose. Sometimes people cannot digest lactose and they get diarrhoea. However, lactose intolerance does not cause eczema.

It is the protein that is the problem. The proteins in cow's milk (whey and casein) can cause allergic reactions. In addition, there is gathering concern about the structure of one of its proteins. This is known as the A1/A2 controversy about beta-casein. There are two main types of milk: A1 and A2, based on the structure this beta-casein protein. The A1 type has been associated with chronic diseases such as heart disease, Type 1 diabetes, autism and schizophrenia. This is too complex to be examined in this book, but it is another reason to be wary of giving your child too much cow's milk.

The make-up of a protein

To help you understand which "milk" you can safely feed your baby, I need to tell you a little more about proteins and how they are made.

Proteins are the molecules, the fundamental substance with which your body's cells are made. Proteins are needed for growth, repair and maintenance of all of your body tissues. A protein molecule can be pictured as a long necklace (a string of beads) that is made up of 20 different sorts of beads. Each of these beads represents an amino acid. Amino acids are the individual building blocks of proteins. Here is a diagram to help you.

Protein (a string of amino acids)

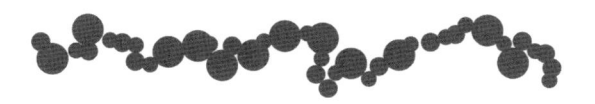

Amino acids are the individual components that make up proteins. There are 20 different amino acids.

Amino acids (separate molecules)

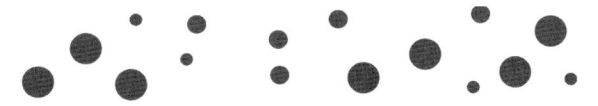

First, here is a collection of individual beads that represent the individual amino acids. You'll have to imagine that there are 20 different types, each standing for one of the 20 different amino acids. All 20 of the amino acids are necessary to build these protein chains. The sequence of how these individual amino acids are strung together determines the type of protein. Peptides are very short chains of amino acids.

As a human, you cannot make all of these amino acids in your body. The ones that you cannot make are called essential amino acids (there are 11 of these). Therefore, you have to get your protein building blocks from your diet. It is crucial for you to eat the right proteins.

Again, a **protein** looks like a long string of beads, like this –

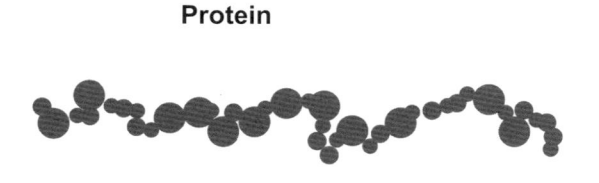

Protein

However, a **peptide** is a very short chain of amino acids. You can make peptides by chopping a protein into small lengths, like this –

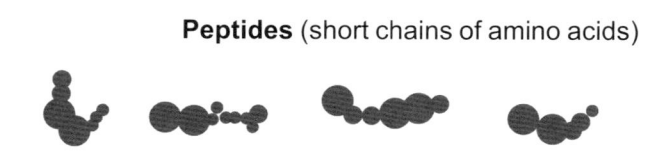

Peptides (short chains of amino acids)

Breast milk is usually the best

Under "normal" circumstances, there is no question that "breast is best" in terms of milk for a baby. Breast milk is the perfect source of food nutrition and immunologic support for your baby. However, adverse reactions to the food allergens that come through mother's breast milk are common triggers for eczema. If there are only a few foods that the mother needs to exclude, this is a relatively easy task.

However, if multiple food allergens are coming through your breast milk and making your baby sick, then sometimes it is necessary to wean onto a low allergen formula. This all depends upon how sick your baby is. With lots of allergens identified as causing the baby harm, then it sometimes seems impossible for mothers to modify their diets successfully and remain well nourished.

What is next-best to breast milk?
The "next-best" alternative to breast milk is "artificial" or "formula" feeding. Formula feeding is not equivalent to breast feeding. A formula is a combination of food components that are manufactured to be as close as possible to the food value of breast milk. At this stage these formulas do not have the biological advantages of breast milk and will never capture the depth of breast feeding.

Cow's milk is not suitable
To make a cow's milk formula, the cow's milk has to be modified to reduce the protein, to increase the lactose, to change the fat content, and to alter the mineral composition. A lot of changes need to be made to make it suitable and safe for a baby! However, a cow's milk based formula still contains unmodified cow's milk proteins. And it is the proteins that make it allergenic.

What are the formula choices?
There are a number of different formulas for feeding milk-allergic babies depending upon the severity, the degree of sensitivity and the availability of these special milks. I have put a symbol next to each type of milk to show whether it is composed of complete proteins, peptides (hydrolysed milk) or amino acids (elemental).

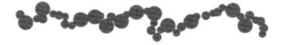

Goat milk formula: made from modified goat's milk and contains goat proteins of casein and whey. Although this suits some children, those who are severely allergic to cow's milk usually react to goat's milk as well. Studies show that up to 90% of children who react to cow's milk will also react to goat's milk proteins.

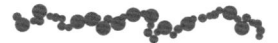

Soy milk formula: made from soy proteins, and all the other nutrients added to make it as similar to breast milk ingredients as practicable. This also suits some children. But again, those who are severely allergic to cow's milk usually react to soy milk as well. Studies show that about 50% of children who react to cow's milk will also react to soy milk. Also, because of the concerns about "phyto-estrogen" in soy, this protein is not recommended for full formula feeding in small babies.

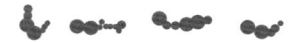

Cow's milk hydrolysates: made from breaking down cow's milk casein or whey into much smaller protein chains, called "peptides". This process greatly reduces the allergic properties of the milk. However, still about 20-30% of children will react adversely to these hydrolysate formulas. Examples of cow's milk hydrolysate formula are *Pepti-Junior* (from whey proteins) and *Pregestimil* (from casein proteins).

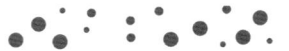

Amino acid formula: created from appropriate mixtures of all 20 amino acids. The other necessary nutrients have been added to make it as similar to the nutrient value of breast milk. There are no peptides or intact proteins in these formulas, therefore they are not allergenic. They are called "elemental" formulas. Examples of amino acid formula are *Neocate and Elecare*.

What some mothers say

As stated above, it turns out that even the extensively hydrolysed milks (such as *Pepti-Junior*) can still upset some children. When that happens, an elemental formula (such as *Neocate*) is required. Here is a mother telling her story of what happened to Joshua when he had extreme eczema at 20 months old with extensive eczema. His mum said:

> "When Joshua had his skin tests, there were strong positive reactions to egg, soy and dairy allergens. Since then, I have seen that all of these foods make his eczema a lot worse if he gets them – and that is only by accidents (for instance, his nana gave him a lick of an ice cream and his eczema flared up terribly in the afternoon)."

> "He went onto the hydrolysed formula *Pepti-Junior* at the time when I was going to wean him off my breast milk. But I just found that he was scratching even worse at night when he had this formula. Especially, he scratched his head – it was bleeding. So we switched to *Neocate* instead. Since then he has not been itching at night at all. His skin is just so much clearer. It's just unbelievable."

Lulu's mother found the same thing. She said:

> "Lulu is now one year old. When she changed to that elemental formula, *Neocate,* she was just a lot happier. She was less whingy, and just generally a happier baby. Her skin was a lot better. Yes! She is a totally different baby and a lot of people have noticed the change in her."

Kyle's mum also has something to say. When he was five months old he had terrible eczema, which had started to develop at about 6 weeks of age. His skin-prick tests were positive to milk. He was being bottle fed with cow's milk formula when I first saw him. Kyle's mum told me:

> "Within a few weeks of changing his formula his skin improved – he was drinking *Pepti-Junior* instead. He would have break outs of his eczema with foods (that contained milk or cheese) scavenged from his older sister. Whenever he has a lick of an ice cream his eczema flares up. He is otherwise fantastic. He is now a happy boy!"

Kyle was 18 months old and his eczema had almost totally disappeared.

The point of these three stories is to emphasize that eczema is frequently caused by cow's milk. Such patients' eczema will not get better until *all* cow milk protein is eliminated from the baby's diet. This means that if mum is breastfeeding, then she needs to take *all* dairy out of her diet. And if the child is formula fed, then it is a matter of finding *exactly* the right formula, which sometimes requires a bit of experimentation.

However, there are other foods that spark off eczema. And *all* of the implicated foods have to be removed before significant improvement will be seen. The next most important food in babies is egg.

Cow's milk is a common eczema trigger

Egg

Egg allergy is one of the most common foods to spark eczema. So many eczema babies have an egg allergy that, in fun, I sometimes call this condition *eggzema*!

It is the egg-white that is such a strong allergen. However, you can also be allergic to the egg-yolk. When a baby is breastfed, these egg proteins readily carry over into the breast milk and can sensitize the baby and this can then trigger eczema.

Most mothers are unaware that the egg they are eating might be harming their child. Initially the baby gets irritable, and then as the weeks go by the baby's face gets rashy. The next step is for the cheeks to become bright red, scaly and dry. Sometimes the skin will crack and weep. The baby begins to rub his cheeks on the bedding which damages the skin even more. The rash continues spreading to the chin, the neck and the creases of the arms and legs. Then the whole body begins to feel rough and a fine red rash appears. This progression occurs over a few weeks to months.

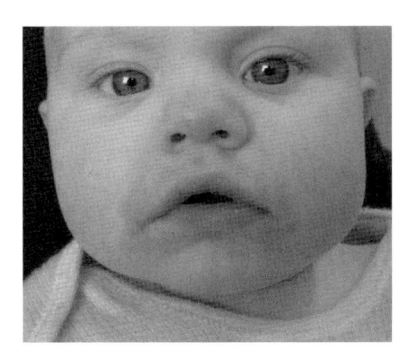

Samantha had bad eczema. At six months old she was still being breast fed. Her mum said:

> "At six weeks of age, she was on the breast and doing fine. But by 12 weeks of age, she seemed to be a bit more hungry, so I introduced a few bottles of some cow's milk formula and her skin felt like blunt sandpaper. She scratches all the time. She scratches until there is blood everywhere. Sometimes her skin is red and patchy, sometimes it clears a bit. As soon as we take her clothes off, she begins to grab her chest and scratch and rub her legs together until they bleed."

"We were told by our doctor that it is quite normal for children to have dry skin. She also had bad cradle cap, and although the hydrocortisone cream does dampen it all down, I am afraid to use it too much."

> "When we got the skin tests done, Samantha showed up positive to milk, egg and peanut. At least I then knew what foods were troubling her. It was a relief to know. After just a few weeks of my staying off these foods, Samantha's skin got so much better. She still has dry scratchy skin, but it is now much easier to manage."

It is my experience that most of these children need to be on a diet that excludes dairy, eggs and peanuts. Alex's mum went on a diet excluding dairy, eggs and peanuts because of Alex's severe eczema. She later said:

> "Yes, there was quite a marked difference in his eczema. His face cleared up really well and he is a lot happier child. He is not scratching anymore and it definitely has made a difference".

Milk, egg and peanut!

Peanut

Peanut allergy has become a serious food allergy that is increasingly common. A large proportion of the children who are allergic to cow's milk or egg are also allergic to peanuts, so it is important to check for peanut allergy in children with eczema, especially if they are being breast fed.

Peanut proteins and peptides can easily travel through the breast milk and affect the baby – the telltale sign is bright, red, scaly, rough cheeks that won't heal. It shows up clinically much like the egg allergy.

Children should not be given peanuts in the first years of life as it is such an allergenic food. Skin-prick testing is an accurate way to pick up a peanut allergy prior to the child being given any.

Allergy children should not be given peanuts

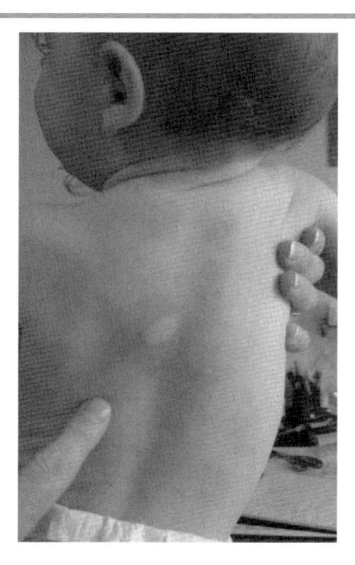

peanut skin-prick test

Gluten

The next chapter deals with the gluten story, which to my thinking is the most exciting part of the eczema story. It begins with a story recounted by Blair in the next chapter. He is thrilled that after 30 years of constant suffering, that his eczema is at last healed. And the cure was simply a gluten-free diet.

I have hundreds of similar stories. One such story is about my daughter, Liz, who was also suffering with eczema. When she read one of my early gluten books she said, "Dad, I think that I have got this gluten thing too!" I organised her blood tests, and yes, she had a high level of IgG-gliadin antibodies. Now that she has been gluten free for the last five years her eczema has gone away - as long as she sticks to her gluten-free diet.

In my audit of children with gluten-sensitivity, a quarter (24%) of these children had eczema. Many of these children also had allergies to other foods (especially cow's milk, eggs and peanuts). Most had good remission of their eczema on a gluten-free diet. The gluten story is told in detail in the next chapter.

In summary

If there is evidence of a food allergy (particularly by skin-prick testing), and if the baby is exclusively breastfed, then it is the mother's role to exclude the implicated food from her diet. This will usually involve removing egg, peanut and perhaps dairy. If these are the problem foods, then the child's skin will dramatically improve within weeks. Often their skin will heal completely. However, these children do have naturally dry and itchy skin, so mild flare-ups may still occur.

Those babies weaned from the breast need to be on an appropriate formula and their parents need to ensure that their diet excludes any of the suspect and high allergenic foods.

6. The Gluten Syndrome!

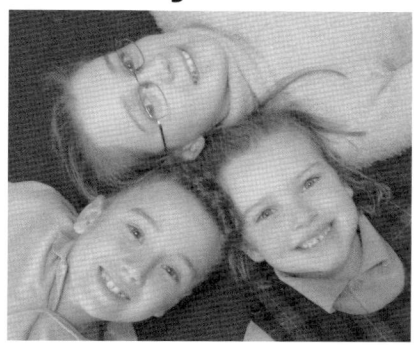

My discovery of the link between gluten and eczema has a large impact on how much I can help my patients with chronic severe eczema. Eczema is often part of the Gluten Syndrome: gluten affecting the nerves, the gut and the skin.

Over the last ten years I have become aware that eating gluten has a major influence on eczema sufferers. I came to this conclusion from doing gluten-antibody blood tests on all of my eczema patients. I found that a large proportion of children with persistent eczema were reacting to gluten. The more children I put on a gluten-free diet, the more success I had with curing their eczema.

Blair is one such person. He was referred to me because of his terrible and unremitting eczema. His skin was itchy everywhere, it was red and angry. He was desperate for help. After just a year he is now completely better. He tells his story below.

Gluten is the major food trigger

Blair's long-awaited recovery

"Hi, my name is Blair, I am 33 years old. I guess it's been a year ago since I was diagnosed with gluten sensitivity."

"I was born with allergies. I developed asthma and eczema when I was six months old, and I pretty much spent most of my younger years, up until about fifteen years old, in and out of hospital with different asthma conditions and skin conditions. But mostly it was eczema that troubled me. Throughout that time I had been given steroid creams, and also prednisone (an oral steroid) to control both my eczema and asthma."

Over the past four years I have had a lot more problems with my skin. It has gone from being eczema, to like a lot of itchy rash all over my body. In these last four years I have seen probably twenty different skin specialists across the country, trying to find a solution to the problem. Everybody has been prescribing me antihistamines, and different types of potent steroids or hydrocortisone creams to try and fix the problem. Some people had looked at different types of foods, but nobody had come up with a cure."

"Over those last four years my skin had got progressively worse – to the point where I really did question my sanity over the whole thing. I was going to bed at night, scratching myself silly (because while you are asleep you don't know you are scratching – but you are!). I would wake up with blood on the sheets and my skin was getting really red and itchy. It was all over my arms, my ribs, my legs, and my back – everywhere!"

"About a year ago, I went and saw Doctor Rodney Ford. He checked me over and listened to my problems. He then did some skin tests and some blood tests on me. A few days later he rang me up and told me that he had found out that I was reacting to gluten. He said that I had a high gluten antibody in my blood (he called it a gliadin antibody). He went on to recommend that I stop eating all gluten based foods. So that meant I had to cut out all wheat, rye and barley... and of course any foods with these in them."

"Of course I was a bit sceptical! I had already seen about twenty other people. But Dr. Rodney Ford was not interested in giving me any more creams. He seemed confident that a gluten-free diet could help."

"It did! Within about four to six weeks of altering my diet, my skin improved noticeably. Over the past year I have found that my skin is getting a lot better because I have become more aware of my diet, what I can eat, what types of food I should avoid."

"I could start to notice it if I ate a gluten-based product, for example a pie, or if I have a pizza or I ate fish and chips (something like that, which contained flour). Within a few hours, and sometimes within six hours, my skin would start to itch again and it would flare up."

"What I have also noticed with this change of diet is that I have previously always suffered with asthma. I have always been very allergic – I am allergic to everything! Be it hay-fever in the summer, dust at people's houses, cats were a killer, and dogs too – it seems just everything irritates me."

"Well, I have found by going onto this gluten-free diet my skin has improved one hundred fold. You know, I still get a little bit of eczema here and there, which I guess is something I have always had. But I really would say that it is a ninety nine percent improvement compared to what it was like before. My other allergies also seem to be going away: I haven't had hay-fever for near on a year when I was previously getting hay-fever two or three times a week."

"My mother made a comment to me a few months ago when she saw the improvements in my skin. She said that maybe over my whole life that gluten might have been the trigger. Maybe the gluten has been the trigger for my whole life and no one has ever understood it or been able to diagnose it."

"So, going off gluten has made a huge improvement to my way of life. Like I say, my skin particularly on my face and my body got to a point where I couldn't control my itching, I became quite embarrassed and quite self conscious because the rash had spread to my neck, my face, my eyelids, all over the place and I really became quite embarrassed about being seen in public, my skin was quite concerning to me."

"So, when I did see Doctor Rodney Ford, I really was at my wits end about what I could do with myself, how to fix it. I had tried so many things, and seen so many different people. But no one had a result or an answer for me."

"He has really made a massive difference to my way of life now, I am pretty happy, no complaints now! My skin has cleaned up, and like I say, my health is back to what I would consider one hundred percent."

"I am very grateful for what he has done, and hopefully this message can be passed on to other people as a means of learning. I guess in some people's view this as an alternative type treatment, but it does work very well if you give it a go and stick it out. Especially, I guess, if you have a positive blood test to gluten."

"I would add that I had been seeing a skin specialist doctor (yes, a dermatologist) for many years. He was a doctor who I went back to time and again for a couple of years with pretty much limited results. He just gave me different steroid creams. He was about to give me his last effort – a very heavy steroid that he said would compromise my immune system. He told me it was a treatment of last resort because I didn't respond to any of his other treatments."

"So, I was very pleased to find out that I didn't have go through that treatment! Obviously, I didn't want to damage my immune system through these treatments. Because a huge improvement happened after I stopped eating gluten, it meant that I didn't have to go down that path. Yes! I am pretty happy about that."

"By the way, when my skin got better off gluten, I decided to go back to my dermatology doctor specialist for a last time. I booked an appointment – I didn't mind paying his fee. I wanted to show him that I had at last got better after thirty years by simply going on this gluten-free diet. I wanted to let him know so that he could help other people like me. But this visit was a big disappointment. He gave me the impression that I was just wasting his time. He didn't seem interested. I think he just put it down to a coincidence. I don't think that he wanted to recognise that my eczema had disappeared with a treatment that he hadn't prescribed. It is just such a pity. I had such a massive improvement in my skin and he just dismissed the concept. That is why I am telling my story. Everyone with eczema needs to know that gluten might be the trigger for their problems."

"If you have got ongoing eczema problems, then why not get tested for gluten?"

Sincerely, Blair H.

Unfortunately, Blair's story is not an isolated incident. Every day I see eczema patients who are getting sick from gluten. Keely is one of these children. Her mum said:

"We were on holiday. Keely is our toddler - she was nearly two years old at the time and she had started her gluten-free diet, because we had discovered that gluten brought her skin out in eczema. She had a positive blood test to gliadin (a test for gluten)."

"Well, because all the other kids had cocktail sausages to eat, we felt a bit mean about this. So we told Keely that she was allowed to eat *just one*. But, when I wasn't looking, Keely had five! Quite quickly she became very itchy and had a sore tummy. I think that she has now learnt her lesson and realizes now that she just can't take these risks. I've noticed that she gets the itching within about an hour of eating the gluten."

Gluten known to cause skin disease

It has been known for a long time that gluten can and does cause skin disease. The classic example is a very itchy rash called "Dermatitis herpetiformis" (DH). It usually affects the elbows, knees, buttocks, scalp, and back. It begins as little bumps that then change into little blisters. People say that they are driven mad by the itching.

> Gluten can cause itchy skin

Dermatitis herpetiformis is caused by an immune reaction to gluten in the skin. Microscopic clumps of gluten (called immune-complexes) get deposited just under the skin. This creates that itchy rash. These tiny particles of gluten can take years to clear up once you start on a gluten-free diet. It may take up to ten years before you make a full recovery.

Humbert and his dermatology colleagues (2006) wrote this about gluten and skin disease:

> "Gluten sensitivity, with or without celiac disease symptoms and intestinal pathology, has been suggested as a potentially treatable cause of various diseases. There have been numerous reports linking celiac disease with several skin conditions. Dermatitis herpetiformis is actually a skin manifestation of celiac disease. Autoimmune diseases, allergic diseases, psoriasis and miscellaneous diseases have also been described with gluten intolerance."

"Dermatologists should be familiar with the appraisal of gluten sensitive enteropathy and should be able to search for an underlying gluten intolerance. Serological screening by means of anti-gliadin, anti-endomysial and tissue-transglutaminase antibodies should be performed. Gluten intolerance gives rise to a variety of dermatological manifestations which may benefit from a gluten-free diet."

This is an important statement. I have discovered that gluten intolerance is very common in children (and adults) with troublesome persistent eczema. It is certainly well worth looking for. Gluten is *the most* common food trigger for eczema.

Gluten can cause eczema

How can you tell if gluten is the problem?

The first thing is to be aware that there actually *is* a link between gluten and eczema. The next step is to get the blood tests. It is crucial to get the appropriate blood tests *before* you think about going on a gluten free diet. There are a number of reasons why I advise this:

1) It is important to get an accurate diagnosis. Eczema can be associated with celiac disease (that is gut damage from gluten), with immune function problems (immuno-deficiencies), with other allergy problems and with nutritional deficiencies. So a full range of blood tests is necessary. The blood tests that I recommend are detailed in the next section.

2) It requires full commitment to the diet for at least six months. All gluten, with no exceptions has to be completely removed from the diet. Having an accurate diagnosis with the appropriate blood tests will help you keep on track. You need to be sure that going gluten-free is the right thing to do.

3) A gluten-free diet, once started and once found beneficial is usually a life-time affair. When gluten is reintroduced, the symptoms can come back with a vengeance. So gluten-free is not something to take up without due consideration.

4) Once you have discovered that your child is gluten sensitive, it is important to look at the whole family. It is likely that other family members will be experiencing gluten symptoms, yet they are often unaware of the cause.

Eczema blood tests

There are a number of blood tests that I recommend. I have written extensively about the gluten tests in my book, "The Gluten Syndrome" – you can access the main content at the website: www.doctorgluten.com. I repeat, do not go gluten-free without first getting your blood tests.

Blood tests help work out the eczema problem

Blood tests recommended for investigating eczema

- **IgG-gliadin** (also called IgG anti-gliadin antibody).
  Looking for immunological response to gluten.

- **IgA-gliadin** (also called IgA anti-gliadin antibody).
  Looking for immunological response to gluten.

- **tTG** (also called IgA tissue transglutaminase antibody).
  Looking for gut damage from gluten (celiac disease).

- **Total IgA** antibody levels.
  Looking for deficiency in your IgA antibody production.

- **Total immunoglobulins.**
  Looking for immuno-deficiency.

- **Total IgE** antibody.
  Looking for the degree of allergic response.

- **Ferritin** (this is a measure of your iron stores).
  Looking for low iron levels.

- **Hb** (Hemoglobin).
  Looking for anaemia.

- **CRP** (called C-Reactive-Protein).
  Looking for evidence of inflammation.

For much more detail about these blood tests and their interpretation you can go to the website:
www.doctorgluten.com

More about gliadin

Gliadin is part of the gluten structure. Gluten is a food protein found in the grains of wheat, rye and barley. This protein has a number of components, one of which is called *gliadin*. It is bad luck that so many people with eczema react to gliadin.

IgG-gliadin (also called IgG anti-gliadin antibody)
The blood test that I am stressing is the IgG-gliadin antibody test. IgG-gliadin is a specific antibody that is made by your immune system when it is assaulted by the gluten that you eat in your diet.

A high level of IgG-gliadin indicates that you do have an immunological response to gluten, and you will most likely develop symptoms from gluten (I suggest that you ask for a copy of your results and look at the numbers for yourself).

My research shows that the IgG-gliadin test is a reliable test for gluten-sensitivity. The majority of people with high IgG-gliadin levels have *The Gluten Syndrome*. However, most do not have coeliac disease.

Check out you laboratory first
Unfortunately, there is a problem. Not all medical laboratories can offer the tests that look for gluten (the IgG-gliadin tests). So you may have to phone a few labs to enquire specifically about whether they can do the gliadin test.

Also, not all laboratories do the same sorts of gluten tests. Different 'antibody kits' are used that give varying results. In my clinic the IgG-gliadin tests are done with test systems manufactured by *Inova Diagnostics*, San Diego, USA.

Ask your lab about their gliadin tests

Gluten eczema stories

To help you get a better idea of how gluten can trigger eczema, here are few more stories of children whose eczema got better when their gluten sensitivity was recognised and treated.

Lily is five years old. She had been diagnosed with celiac disease. All of her blood tests were positive for celiac disease and she had an abnormal intestinal biopsy which confirmed the bowel damage of celiac disease. Also, she had very high gluten antibody levels. Her mum said:

> "Lily has now been gluten-free for the last year. She came to see Dr. Ford because of her allergies. She had a blocked nose and troublesome eczema. She had quite a pot tummy and had slow growth. She had blood tests for gluten and celiac disease: these were both positive. So she had an endoscopy, which again was positive showing that she had celiac disease. Therefore, she went gluten-free."

> "Since she has been gluten-free over the last year, she has gotten better and better. She no longer has lots of infections, she has more energy, and interestingly, her allergies have nearly gone away. Her skin used to give her a lot of trouble – she had a lot of bad eczema. Her eczema now is very much better and she only has small amounts left in her creases. And if she has any gluten errors it flares up."

Gluten errors cause flares ups

Isabella, at two years old, was recovering from her eczema. I asked her mother what happens if Isabella has any gluten. Her mum said:

> "Isabella had eczema all over her body. She was on strong steroid creams. She had the positive blood tests for gluten antibodies, so it was suggested I take her off the gluten. I did this. I took her off gluten and it has cleared her eczema up. Now, when she does eat anything with gluten in it she gets little patches of eczema on her legs. I just can't believe it!"

Gluten is a leading cause of eczema

Emily was three years old. She had a high IgG-gliadin antibody test but she did not have coeliac disease. Her mother told me:

> "Initially her skin was really sore, dry and scratchy. She would have blood all over her sheets in the morning from scratching while she was asleep. Her poos were really sloppy and nasty. But after taking gluten out of her diet her skin cleared up within days, and the itchiness of her skin settled. She was just so much happier."

Think about the gluten-eczema link

Yes! Gluten is an important trigger for eczema.

Think about it. Test for it. Treat it.

My research findings show that the majority of people over three years of age, who have ongoing and troublesome eczema, have a gluten-sensitivity. When gluten is removed from their diets, they get better. Advice about blood testing for gluten and for information on a gluten-free diet can be found on our webpage: www.doctorgluten.com

---
Gluten is the hidden culprit

"Every truth passes through three stages before it is recognized.
In the first, it is ridiculed,
In the second, it is opposed,
In the third, it is regarded as self-evident."

Arthur Schopenhauser

7. Eczema! Switch it off!

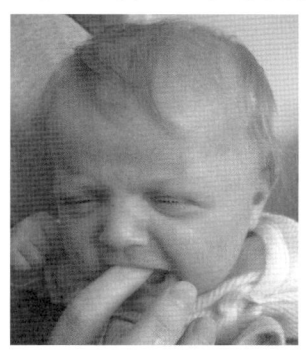

An intriguing and crucial advance in the treatment and management of eczema is the understanding of probiotics. They can switch off your eczema. Also, you might be able to prevent your future children from ever getting eczema in the first place.

Good gut bugs

The term "probiotic" is used to describe the good bugs (healthy bacteria) in your gut. Your colon (that is the last part of your bowel) is teaming with bacteria. These bacteria carry out vital functions in your gut, living in harmony with you. At birth your gut is sterile; there are no bacteria in your gut when you are in the womb.

However, as soon as you are born, you come into contact with the outside world. Immediately you get bacteria coating your skin and the insides of your gut. You should get these bugs from your mother as you roll on her skin and swallow some of the fluids from the birth canal as you exit the uterus. These bacteria should be the "good" bacteria that help protect you from getting sick. These good bugs will displace the "bad" (harmful) bacteria.

It has been discovered that having the right types of bacteria is crucial for your immune system's health. It seems that the right bacteria in your gut, soon after birth, make a big difference to whether you will develop allergies as you grow.

The allergy "switch" theory

It seems that all babies are born with the potential to develop allergies. While they are growing in the womb they go into an "allergy" mode. Metaphorically, they have a sort of "allergy switch". If this is left "on", then this new born baby will go down the allergy path. But if this switch can be turned "off", then the baby will avoid developing allergies in the future. Naturally, we all want this allergy switch turned "off".

Here are a few more details about this theory. This so called "allergy switch" is thought to come about by the incompatibility of immune systems between the growing fetus (the baby) and the mother. The scenario goes as follows.

When the mother conceives, and the baby begins to grow in her womb, mother and baby have different tissue-types to one another (this is because the baby has genes from both father and mother). This is the crux of the problem: this mismatch of tissue types.

As a result, the mother's immune system begins attempting to reject this new "foreign object" (the baby) from her womb. However, the baby, who desperately wants to stay on in the womb and fully develop, fights back. This creates a tug-of-war which the baby happily wins. But the cost of this war is the possibility of future allergy. The "allergy switch" needs to be turned off.

The allergy switch turns "on"

To stay in the womb, it seems that the baby generates a sort of allergic response against the mother. This allergic reaction helps the baby overcome the mother's immune mechanism. This allows the baby to remain safe. But the cost of this strategy is that at birth, the baby is in an "allergy mode".

Bugs can turn eczema off

Now back to the probiotics, the good bugs in your gut. The types of bacteria that colonize your colon in the first few hours of life seem to be critical to what happens to this "allergy switch". In some mysterious way, these probiotic bacteria communicate to the immune system through the mucosa of the colon. Their chemical message seems to switch off the allergic mechanism. If this switching off does not occur, then the baby might develop eczema.

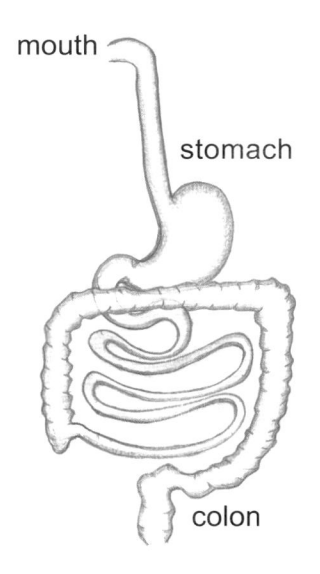

Probiotics can stop eczema

The title "Probiotics in the management of atopic eczema" was used for one of the earliest papers that presented the evidence that probiotics could be important in the treatment of baby eczema. This was reported by Isolauri and colleagues (2000). They studied 27 babies. They were five months old and all had bad eczema and were exclusively breast fed.

They were randomly divided into three groups: the first group was given the probiotic *Bifidobacterium lactis*, the second group was given the probiotic *Lactobacillus GG;* and the third group were given a *placebo*. They were also put on a cow's milk free diet - they were weaned onto an extensively hydrolysed whey formula (*Pepti-junior*).

After two months, they saw a big improvement in their eczema. They claimed that this was the first clinical demonstration that probiotics, fed to babies with eczema, could modify the allergic inflammation. They went on to say that these probiotic strains could protect infants through the weaning period, when sensitization to newly encountered antigens is initiated. They believed that probiotics had the potential for food allergy treatment and allergy prevention in the future. Since this study, other research has confirmed these findings.

Probiotics can prevent eczema

Not only can eczema be cured with the assistance of probiotics, but now evidence also suggests that it can be prevented: simply by giving probiotics from birth.

If there is a strong family history of eczema, then early feeding with probiotics can prevent eczema. If the mother is given probiotics in the last trimester of pregnancy and the child given probiotics from the day of birth, then the chance of eczema ever developing is halved.

This work was carried out by Viljanen and colleagues (2005). In this study they documented the severity of eczema in 230 babies with suspected cow's milk allergy. These children were given a mixture of four probiotic strains of *lactobacillus* bacteria, or placebo (a dummy treatment) for four weeks. In addition, they were put on an elimination diet (that is no cow's milk protein, eggs or nuts). They were also given appropriate skin treatment.

Four weeks after this probiotic treatment, cow's milk allergy was diagnosed using the double-blind placebo-controlled technique. This "milk challenge" showed that 120 infants had milk allergy.

Their final results were interesting. For the whole group, they found a 65% improvement in their eczema. But in the IgE-sensitized infants (that is those with a positive skin-prick test to cow's milk), the probiotic group showed an even greater improvement in their eczema. They concluded that treatment with probiotics may alleviate atopic eczema symptoms in IgE-sensitized infants.

How do probiotics work?

Research has now clearly demonstrated the preventive and curative effects of probiotics in allergy patients. Adequate doses of probiotics have been shown to have the following effects:

- Prevent the increased intestinal permeability (leaky gut) of children with atopic eczema and food allergy.
- Prevent the uptake of food allergens from the gut into the bloodstream.
- Prevent the actual development (or expression) of the atopic condition.
- Reduce amounts of the bacterial, toxic metabolites in the intestine.
- Promote the gut barrier function.
- Stimulate local release of interferon, improving immunity.
- Prevent unfavourable bacterial alterations of the intestines in allergic children.

Some probiotics, although not all, appear to exert beneficial effects by enhancing the mucosal barrier function of the gut and stimulating immune activity. It seems that a combination of different probiotics is more effective than a single strain.

Summary

The message seems clear. Probiotics are essential for good immunity. They are a big leap forward in the treatment of eczema. Children developing eczema have relatively low levels of acidophilus and other probiotics.

If probiotics are given to children on a daily basis: their gut health improves; their immune health improves; and the inflammatory activity in their skin is reduced. Current recommendations are to give probiotics to:

- Mothers during the third trimester of pregnancy.
- Babies with a family history of allergies.
- Reduce allergic diseases, including eczema, from day one through to at least the first year of life.
- Babies and children with eczema who have positive skin tests.

Studies show that regular probiotics can improve most babies with troublesome eczema. In combination with the appropriate exclusion of problematic foods, and skin care, many of these children should be cured of their eczema.

Now it is time to look at skin care.

Good bugs help in lots of ways

8. Creams and potions!

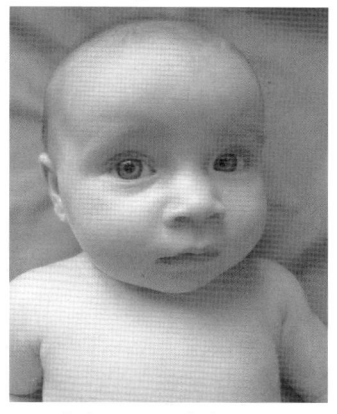

Skin care is an essential part of the management of someone with eczema. People who have eczema have irritable and dry skin. I call it "twitchy" skin, because all manner of things can cause a flare-up. Creams and potions do have an important place. This is a brief overview of strategies that are available to give your skin the daily care it needs.

Soaps

No soap! Generally, soap should be avoided. This is because washing with soap removes the natural oils from skin. Soap will dry out skin even more, and makes the whole situation worse.

Moisturizers and oils

Moisturisers are also called "emollients". These are used to help stop skin from drying out. Even when your skin is looking and feeling good it is still a good idea to use a moisturiser every day. These come in the form of lotions, creams, ointments and bath/shower additives. These can certainly help oil your skin and prevent your skin from drying out and cracking. They help keep your skin feeling moist and smooth.

Steriods

"Topical steroids" are steroid creams that are rubbed onto skin. Usually, steroid creams and ointments are prescription medicines. Steroid medications are very effective at calming down inflammation – but unfortunately they have troublesome side effects.

Advice for using topical steroids

Topical steroids creams and ointments are absorbed at different rates from different parts of the body. A steroid that works on your face (which is very delicate skin) might not work on your palm or foot (which is tough skin). A potent steroid may be good for tough skin, but it would quickly cause side effects on your face. Consequently, it is very important to know the strengths of the steroid creams that you are using. Another problem is that your skin can become accustomed to these steroid creams with prolonged use. These creams are best used in intermittent bursts.

Check out the "potency"

These steroid creams can be grouped according to their strength or "potency". The general rule is to use the least potent steroid, for the shortest time. The stronger the cream, the more quickly it will work, but the side effects will be more pronounced.

The table below lists the steroid creams by their potency class. Trade names are given in brackets. They are listed from the mildest (Class 4) to the most potent (Class 1). Both "generic" names and "trade names" are given. A generic name is the general or chemical name for the product. However, each manufacturer also gives their product their own "trade name". Availability varies in different countries. Also, new products are always being developed and put on the market.

Creams and potions!

Please check the prescription that you are using against this list.

Mild steroids (Class 4)

All other classes are compared to this class– hydrocortisone.
    Hydrocortisone 0.5–2.5%

Moderate steroids (Class 3)

These are between **2–20** times more potent than hydrocortisone.
Clobetasone butyrate	(Eumovate)
Triamcinolone acetonide	(Astrocort)

Potent steroids (Class 2)

These are about **50** times more potent than hydrocortisone.
Betamethasone valerate	(Betnovate, Beta cream)
Betamethasone dipropionate	(Diprosone)
Diflucortolone valerate	(Nerisone)
Hydrocortisone 17-butyrate	(Locoid)
Mometasone furoate	(Elecon)
Methylprednisolone aceponate	(Advantan)

Very potent steroids (Class 1)

These are around **100** times more potent than hydrocortisone.
Clobetasol propionate	(Dermol)
Betamethasone dipropionate	

Side effects of topical steroids

The risk of any side effects is related to a combination of: the strength of the steroid; the length of time it is used; and the sensitivity of the skin. For example, using a mild cream on your hands or feet for years and years may cause no problems. But using a very potent cream on your face can produce skin problems in just a couple of weeks.

Side effects on your skin:
o   Skin thinning, tearing of the skin.
o   Stretch marks, easy bruising.
o   Prominent blood vessels.
o   Likelihood of skin infections.
o   Allergic reactions to the cream.

Side effects on your insides:
o   Reduced production of natural steroids.
o   Some fluid retention.
o   Contribute to high blood sugar and diabetes.
o   Raised blood pressure.

Oral steroids
Sometimes, if the eczema gets too bad, then under your doctor's guidance, you might be prescribed a short course of oral steroids. This is started when topical steroids are not working. Again, the smallest dose for the shortest time is the rule. This usually means a seven to ten day course, reducing the dose every couple of days. Oral steroids can quickly cause troublesome side effects.

Find the triggers and reduce steroid use

Non-steroid anti-inflammatory creams

Recently, a couple of "anti-inflammatory" creams have been developed that are not based on steroids. Currently, there are two preparations available: "pimecrolimus" (trade name, *Elidel*) and tacrolimus (trade name, *Protopic Ointment*). They work by suppressing inflammation. This class of medication is known as a "calcineurin inhibitor", also called a "selective cytokine inhibitor". They are prescription medications (they are not available in all countries). The advantage of these calcineurin inhibitors over topical steroids is that they do not cause any skin thinning, or any ocular side effects. This makes them especially useful for delicate skin such as the face: where skin thinning can develop quickly. If this medication is rubbed on at the first signs and symptoms, then it can prevent the progression of the eczema flaring up. It also can reduce the severity of flares. In addition, this medication has been found to reduce the need for topical steroids.

Cancer risk?
However, there is a current health warning about their use. This is because in rare cases, patients have had cancer (e.g. skin or lymphoma) during treatment with these topical calcineurin inhibitors. However, a causal link has not been demonstrated. Nevertheless, caution is necessary with the use of this medication (as in the case with all drugs, including steroids). The concern has been that in animal studies, when these medications have been used at very high *systemic* (not topical) doses, both agents may be associated with the development of skin cancers and lymphomas. The short-term data on systemic side effects for tacrolimus and pimecrolimus is reassuring. Also systemic absorption is low in a majority of patients. But, as cancers take years to develop, the long-term safety data are incomplete. So it will take another decade before enough data is available to document an association, if any, between the use of topical tacrolimus and pimecrolimus and the occurrence of cancer.

Recommendations
These drugs are recommended only for use as second-line treatments. This means that they should be used only after topical steroids have been tried. They are intended for short use. However, if you require a longer period of treatment, the creams can be repeated after a period of time off treatment. Use the minimum amount of pimecrolimus and tacrolimus that are needed to control the symptoms. Continuous long-term use of topical calcineurin inhibitors in any age group should be avoided. Their application should also be limited just to the areas of eczema.

Also, they should be restricted to patients who are over two years old. If used in babies, applications should be limited to the smallest practicable areas. It is my policy to use tiny amounts on the face and only if the eczema remains troublesome. Such treatment should generally be limited to no more than three weeks. These drugs may be used as an alternative to or in combination with topical steroids, but their use should be carefully monitored and patients' responses should be followed closely.

Antiseptics and antibiotics

Local application of antiseptics can reduce the chance of the eczema getting infected. Unfortunately, eczema does often become infected. When this happens, the skin can be weepy and will not heal. Under these circumstances, the skin needs treatment with appropriate antibiotics to kill the infecting bacteria. Sometimes antibiotics are needed for several months.

Antihistamines

An "antihistamine" is a medication that reduces the effects of the chemical histamine. When histamine is released in the skin it causes bad itching. Anti-histamines can reduce the itching, especially in the very allergic child. Some antihistamines cause drowsiness as well.

9. Eczema! Prevent it!

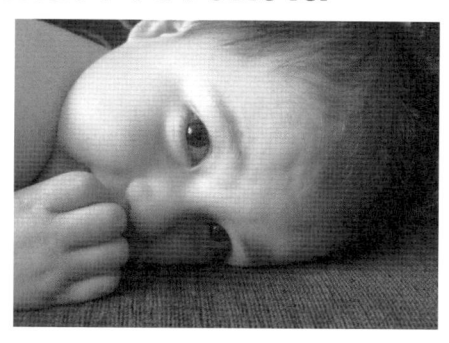

Surely, the very best way to manage eczema is to avoid getting it in the first place! This means stopping eczema before it ever starts. Yes! Prevent it!

Eczema Prevention Strategy

This is now a possibility, but you have to start early. This *Eczema Prevention Strategy* is a matter of taking everything that you have learned so far, and putting it into action in preparation for your next baby.

It is my clinical experience that most allergies can be cured. It is all about doing the right thing at the right time. The most crucial time is during pregnancy and the first few months of life. Preventing eczema is all about the identification of foods that cause eczema, the improvement of the immune system, and dampening down the allergic responses.

Each of the following ten steps in the *Eczema Prevention Strategy* is important. This is because eczema is a step-by-step process, each building on the next, slowly but surely leading to established eczema - unless the process can be halted. The earlier that you can start on the prevention process, the better will be your results. There are ten steps to take.

Ten steps to prevent eczema

1. Before pregnancy: diet.
2. During pregnancy: diet.
3. Birth: probiotics.
4. Infant feeding: breast feeding.
5. Skin tests: early identification.
6. What formula? hydrolysed cow's milk, or amino acid formula.
7. Avoid food allergens: cow's milk, eggs, peanuts, fish, gluten.
8. Avoid inhalant allergens: house dust mites.
9. Antihistamines: Cetirizine.
10. Supplements and skin care.

These are the secrets to preventing and curing eczema. The supporting evidence for these recommendations is given in the previous chapters. A key message is given for each step.

1. Before pregnancy: diet

Good nutrition before pregnancy is important. Heaps of information shows that the healthiest babies are from the healthiest mothers. To be a healthy mother it is very important to be on an appropriate intake of vitamins, minerals and nutrients. This can be achieved through diet and supplements.

The better nourished you are the better nourished your baby is and the better health your baby will have. Eating well, especially lots of fruits and vegetables, is essential. It is also important to be taking a daily supplement of the vitamin "folate" (or folic acid) that reduces the risk of neurological damage to your growing baby.

> **Key message**: Make excellent food choices and take vitamin supplements prior to pregnancy.

2. During pregnancy: diet

During your pregnancy, continue to eat a healthy diet. Surprisingly, there is no need to be on a restricted or "allergy elimination" diet.

The research evidence (much from Warner) shows that going on a food elimination diet during pregnancy does *not* prevent asthma or eczema in your future child. They carried out a seven year follow up study of combined maternal and infant dietary avoidance. The food allergen avoidance diets failed to modify atopic disease at seven years of age, compared with the infant feeding practices customarily followed.

The best advice is to eat in moderation. Of course you need to eat lots of fruit and vegetables and get enough iron and calcium and vitamins and minerals. But going strictly off egg, or peanut, does not reduce the chances of egg and peanut allergy in your child's future.

For the last three months of pregnancy, it is important for you to be on a probiotic. The details are given in the previous chapter. Having a healthy bowel helps you with your own health and it enables you to pass on these good probiotic bugs to your child during the birth.

> **Key message**: Make excellent food choices and take vitamin supplements during pregnancy. Elimination diets do not help at this stage.

Always eat well – every mouthful matters

---

3. Birth: probiotics

Start on day one! The first minutes of your baby's life are crucial. Your baby comes out of your womb sterile. That means that there are no bacteria on the skin or in the gut.

However, as soon as your baby comes into this world, that is the time for the skin to be colonised by bacteria. It is important that the first bacteria your baby is exposed to are from *you*. During the actual delivery, your baby should be inoculated from the bacteria from your birth canal and from your colon. These are the good bugs that you are in tune with (they have been living inside you harmlessly for decades).

Your immune system has made antibodies against these bugs. You will be passing these antibodies on to your baby through your breast milk. So when your baby drinks your breast milk your baby is protected from these gut organisms. These bacteria should be swallowed by your baby and get into the colon and colonize the lower bowel. The colon colonization of your baby is vital to help "switch off" the allergic mechanism.

Your baby also needs skin-to-skin contact with you immediately after birth. Your baby needs to get the bacteria from your skin onto its skin. Having the right skin bacteria is very important for your baby's health. Also, there are chemicals that you are excreting through your skin pores and through your breast milk. There is a "chemical attraction" between you and your baby which helps with breastfeeding and bonding.

> **Key message**: Take a high quality probiotic during the third trimester of pregnancy. Give your baby a probiotic from day one through to at least the first year of life. Make sure that the probiotic is free of dairy and gluten.

4. Infant feeding: breast feeding

Your baby needs to be suckled on the breast as soon as possible. This gives the magic colostrum to your baby, which is very important for the "immune priming" of your baby's immune system. This colostrum is full of good antibodies that your baby can absorb whole. Shortly after birth, the baby's stomach acid is weak. Also, in the first few days of life your baby's gut is more "leaky". This allows the antibodies from your breast milk to get into your baby's immune system.

This mechanism also allows other harmful food allergens in as well. Therefore, at this stage it is best for you to start your elimination diet avoiding egg and peanut. You may also want to avoid dairy. Gluten can also be problematic at this time.

The best food for your baby is breast milk. Breast milk contains a whole range of wonderful nutritional and immunological benefits. It is best to exclusively breast feed your baby through to at least six months. This helps your child avoid other food allergens. The data shows that the later that your baby is exposed to food allergens, the less likely a food allergy and eczema will develop.

You can have soy or protein-enriched rice milk instead of dairy. Of course it is important that while you are breastfeeding you have an adequate calcium intake.

Breast feed if you can

If you choose to formula feed your child, then the recommendation is for a partially hydrolysed formula (different countries have different brands of these milks: such as *Karicare HA*). Medical evidence shows that soy formula feeding is not preventive of allergies. I do not recommend soy formula for babies.

Allergic sensitisation of a baby to food proteins has been shown to occur through the breast milk in about 5% of high-risk infants. But there is good news for mothers who exclusively breastfeed: if you restrict cow's milk, egg, fish, peanut and soy in your own diet, then you can substantially reduce the chance of eczema in your child.

> **Key message**: Low allergen diets in mothers who are breast-feeding high-risk infants can reduce the chance of that child developing eczema in early life.

5. Food skin-prick tests: early identification

If your baby does develop eczema in the first few months, I recommend skin-prick testing to check for any sensitivity to common food allergens.

These tests are best done at about three months. Test for: cow's milk, egg white, peanut, soy and wheat. If positive, then exclude these foods from mother's and hence, the baby's diet. This might require a special formula.

I recommend food and inhalant allergen skin-prick testing again at 1 year, 2 years and 5 years of age.

> **Key message**: skin prick testing is essential to identify trigger allergens early in life. Avoidance of these allergenic foods substantially reduces eczema.

Prevent it!

6. What formula?

Breastfeed for as long as you can. Give breast milk only to 6 months of age and, if possible, keep breastfeeding to 12 months. However, if you have to exclude multiple foods from your diet, then it might be too difficult for you to breastfeed long term.

Formula technology has come a long way. Artificial milk formulas have an important role. However, the decision about how to feed a new baby is not a menu choice. Formula feeding is not bio-equivalent to breast feeding.

When it comes time to offer a formula, avoid cow's milk proteins. That means using a cow's milk hydrolysate (such as *Pepti-Junior*) or an amino acids based formula (such as *Neocate*) for babies with severe multiple food allergy. These special formulas are expensive. In most countries these formulas require specialist Paediatrician approval.

Soy and goat milk formulas have only a limited place in the management of eczema babies.

> **Key message**: avoid cow's milk formulas. Use a cow's milk hydrolysate or an amino acids based formula for babies with severe multiple food allergy. In most countries these special formulas will need Paediatric specialist approval.

Avoid cow's milk proteins

7. Foods: cows milk, eggs, peanuts, fish, gluten

Late introduction of solids is recommended. This means no solid foods until your baby is six months old. The earlier solids are introduced, and the wider the range of solids, the greater the likelihood that eczema will develop.

When you start solids, it is good to use low allergen foods such as: pear, rice, maize (corn), apples, bananas, avocados, and pumpkin; the root vegetables of potato, kumara (sweet potato), carrot and parsnip; the meats of chicken and lamb; and any leafy vegetable is fine.

Various Paediatric guidelines recommend that you delay the introduction of dairy until 12 months of age; eggs until 24 months of age; and peanuts, tree nuts, fish, and shellfish until 36 months of age.

Gluten. I also recommend avoiding gluten through to 12 months of age. Past a year of age, gluten plays an increasing role in the development of eczema. Often, as the allergic effects of cow's milk and egg are waning, the gluten reaction kicks in. Blood tests for gluten antibodies (IgG-gliadin) can help make this diagnosis. My studies have shown that the majority of troublesome eczema, past three years of age, is triggered by gluten. These children respond very well to a gluten-free diet, but it can take up to six months for the skin to fully recover.

> **Key message**: be aware of any foods that may cause an outbreak and avoid those foods. Skin tests and blood tests can help guide you.

Gluten is an major food allergen

Prevent it!

8. Avoid inhalant allergens: house dust mite.

At 12 months of age I recommend skin-prick testing for inhalant allergens (also called aero allergens). Test for: dust mite, ryegrass, birch pollen, cat fur and dog hair. It can be difficult to avoid these allergens. However dust mites can easily be avoided by using dust mite covers for the bedding. I recommend this from early on (even the baby bassinette mattress). The reduction of dust mite exposure can also reduce the chance of asthma.

If there is an allergic reaction to dust mites, grass pollens, or cat fur, then I would recommend that the child go on an 18 month treatment of Cetirizine.

> **Key message**: past one year pay attention to inhalant allergens. Use dust mite covers over mattresses and pillows. Avoids cats and dogs if possible.

9. Antihistamines: cetirizine

Help reduce itch. An antihistamine is a medication that reduces the action of histamine in the body. Histamine is a chemical that is released from the allergy cells (mast cells) in your skin that causes intense itching. Itch is the predominant feature of atopic eczema. High levels of histamine have been measured in the blood and skin of eczema patients at times of acute exacerbations of their eczema. The chemical histamine can cause intense itching so an antihistamine would seem to be a prefect treatment for eczema.

Antihistamines are also called H^1-antagonists. The medical literature shows a definite anti-pruritic affect of non-sedating antihistamines. Their sedative affect is not connected with the anti-itch affect. *Cetirizine* has also been shown to inhibit eosinophil activity, which are blood cells that play an important part in the allergic mechanism.

Eczema! Cure It!

Help prevent subsequent asthma. You can reduce the chance of eczema babies getting asthma. The *Early Treatment of the Atopic Child* (ETAC) study is a multi-country double blind randomised placebo controlled trial. Over 800 children, aged between 1 and 2 years old, were studied. The children in the study had severe eczema, but had not yet developed asthma. They all had positive skin-prick tests to grass pollens or dust mites. These children were treated with cetirizine (*Zyrtec*), 0.25 mg/kg twice daily, or a placebo.

Only a third of the cetirizine treated group developed asthma compared to two thirds of the placebo group. Giving cetirizine for 18 months (from the age of one year) reduced the chance of developing asthma by 50% - a huge reduction.

Also, encouragingly, the long term use of cetirizine showed beneficial effects in the treatment of eczema by reducing the amount of steroid creams needed. Importantly, cetirizine treatment was shown to be safe.

> **Key message**: eczema children with dust mite and/or grass pollen sensitivity benefit from treatment with cetirizine for 18 months: this will halve the risk of developing asthma later.

Work on reducing the itch
---

10. Supplements and skin care

Vitamins, minerals, essential oils

Inflamed skin is healing skin. To heal, the skin needs all of the vitamins, minerals, and building blocks for new cells. These children are usually on elimination diets. It is essential that they eat everything they need to keep their skin and immune system in top health. This means a fully nourishing diet along with supplements of vitamins, minerals, and essential oils.

> **Key message**: give a high quality vitamin-mineral supplement as well as essential oils.

Soaps, creams, sunscreen

Daily and regular skin care is important. Use emollients/moisturisers several times a day. Protect your child's skin against the sun – use a low allergen sunscreen.

Use topical steroids when needed, and use the weakest preparation that works for the shortest time practical.

Keep temperatures as steady as practicable, try to avoid sudden changes. Reduce sweating and overheating if possible.

Avoid: soaps; irritating clothing such as wool; strong cosmetics; cleaning chemicals such as chlorine or solvents; dust or sand; and cigarette smoke.

> **Key message**: cleanse, moisturise and calm the skin. Use steroid creams to reduce inflammation when necessary.

Final words

Eczema affects millions of people, some only mildly but others can have severe problems. Although there is a great deal that you can do to reduce the burden of eczema, the nature of eczema is to intermittently flare up and then calm down. Happily, for many it can be cured.

If you have eczema, your skin will get itchy from time to time. However, by following the steps of this *eczema prevention strategy* you should find your skin feeling a lot more comfortable. The longer that you persist with these steps, the more your skin will improve.

Please contact me through the webpage to tell your story and to help encourage others who are also on this eczema journey.

www.doctoreczema.com

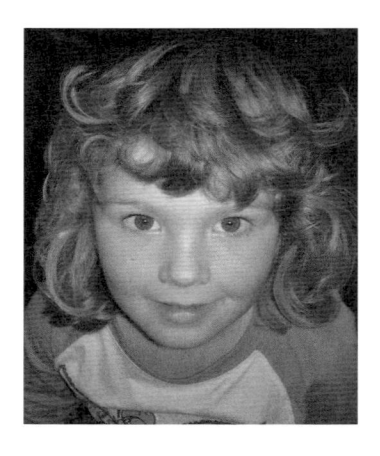

References

This list of references is to acquaint you with some of the history and the names of some of the medical teams who have been part of the research into the relationships between foods and eczema. I have referred to many of these in the previous chapters. A full listing of all of the relevant papers would require hundreds of pages.

American Academy of Dermatology statement:
http://www.skincarephysicians.com/eczemanet/index.html

Atherton DJ, Sewell M, Soothill JF et al.
A double-blind controlled crossover trial of an antigen avoidance diet in atopic eczema. Lancet 1978; I: 401–3.

Diepgen TL; Early Treatment of the Atopic Child Study Group. Long-term treatment with cetirizine of infants with atopic dermatitis: a multi-country, double-blind, randomized, placebo-controlled trial (the ETAC trial) over 18 months. Pediatr Allergy Immunol. 2002; 13: 278–86.

Ford RPK, Fergusson D.
Egg and cow's milk allergy in children.
Arch Dis Child. 1980; 55: 608–610.

Ford RPK, Hill DJ, Hosking CS.
Cow's milk hypersensitivity : immediate and delayed onset clinical patterns.
Arch Dis Child. 1983; 58: 856–862.

Guillet G, Guillet MH. Natural history of sensitizations in atopic dermatitis. A 3-year follow-up in 250 children: food allergy and high risk of respiratory symptoms.
Arch Dermatol.1992; 128: 187–192.

Hill DJ, Ford RPK, Sheldon MJ, Hosking CS.
A study of 100 infants and young children with cow's milk allergy Clinical Reviews in Allergy. 1984; 2: 125–142.

Humbert P, Pelletier F, Dreno B, Puzenat E, Aubin F.
Gluten intolerance and skin diseases. Review.
Eur J Dermatol. 2006; 16: 4–11.

Isolauri E, Arvola T, Sütas Y, Moilanen E, Salminen S.
Probiotics in the management of atopic eczema.
Clin Exp Allergy. 2000; 30:1604–10.

Jakobsson I, Lindberg T. Cow's milk proteins cause infantile colic in breast-fed infants: a double-blind crossover study. Pediatrics. 1983; 71: 268–71.

Lothe L, Lindberg T. Cow's milk whey protein elicits symptoms of infantile colic in colicky formula-fed infants: a double-blind crossover study. Pediatrics. 1989; 83: 262–6.

Mari A, Ballmer-Weber BK, Vieths S. The oral allergy syndrome: improved diagnostic and treatment methods.
Curr Opin Allergy Clin Immunol. 2005; 5: 267–73.

Viljanen M, Savilahti E, Haahtela T, Juntunen-Backman K, Korpela R, Poussa T, Tuure T, Kuitunen M.
Probiotics in the treatment of atopic eczema/dermatitis syndrome in infants: a double-blind placebo-controlled trial.
Allergy. 2005; 60: 494–500.

Warner JO. Early life nutrition and allergy.
Early Hum Dev. 2007; 83:777–83.

Warner JO. The hygiene hypothesis.
Pediatr Allergy Immunol. 2003; 14:145–6.
J Clin Gastroenterol. 2004; 38: 642-5.

Other books by Dr Rodney Ford

☐ Eczema! Cure It!

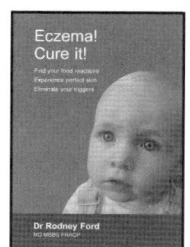

Parents want a cure for their child's eczema! For most, I can help them get their skin back to almost perfect. Find out the secrets! All the information offered in this book is from well-researched approaches to allergy and eczema. Learn how these strategies can help cure your child's eczema. Yes! Eczema can be cured! Find out how!

ISBN 978-0-473-10773-4 (96 pages)
(NZ$24.95 Aus$24.95 US$15.95)

☐ The Gluten Syndrome

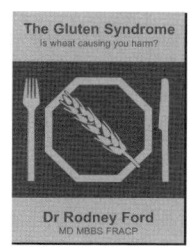

The Gluten Syndrome is the name for the cluster of symptoms that you get when you react to gluten – it can affect your gut, skin and nerves. One in ten people – tens of millions worldwide – are affected but few are aware of this illness. Could this be you?

ISBN 978-0-473-12472-4 (192 pages)
(NZ$34.95 Aus$34.95 US$19.95)

☐ Going Gluten-Free: How to Get Started

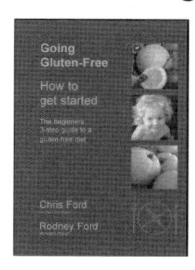

"Overwhelm" is often the first emotion felt when you are confronted by the prospect of a gluten-free diet. Find out how you can get started. Step 1– Get ready: Identify if you really are gluten-sensitive. Step 2 – Get set up: Find out all about gluten. Use our shopping list to help you work out what you can eat. Step 3 – Go gluten-free: Follow the recipes and eating ideas.

ISBN 978-0-473-10491-7 (64 pages)
(NZ$14.95 Aus$14.95 US$9.95)

Available from the website: www.doctorgluten.com

☐ Are You Gluten-Sensitive? Your Questions Answered

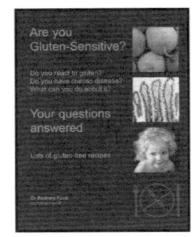

This book is based on the questions that I am so frequently asked by my patients. I answer their questions in detail and put them into the clinical context. There is lots of confusion about the diagnosis and management of people who are gluten-sensitive. This book has been written to clarify this muddle. It is full of practical information.

ISBN 978-0-473-11229-5 (192 pages)
(NZ$34.95 Aus$34.95 US$19.95)

☐ The Gluten-Free Lunch Book

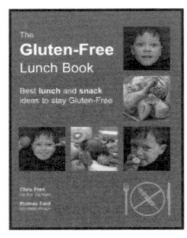

What can I have for lunch? That is our most often asked question. Easy and yummy lunches make all the difference if you are trying to stay gluten-free. We have brought together the best lunch ideas so that you never have to worry about lunch again. Simple and delicious gluten-free lunch box ideas for you and your family. Follow these recipes and eating ideas for a great gluten-free experience.

ISBN 978-0-473-10498-6 (64 pages)
(NZ$14.95 Aus$14.95 US$9.95)

☐ The book for the **Sick, Tired & Grumpy**

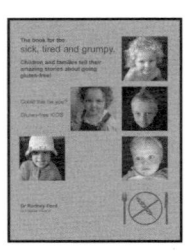

Over 50 people tell their amazing stories. A cure for so many people who feel sick, tired or grumpy. These personal accounts are very moving with a raw honesty that hits home. If you want to feel well and full of energy again – then this book is for you. These children and parents tell about their low energy, their irritability and troublesome symptoms before they discovered their gluten-sensitivity. You then hear how going gluten-free has changed their lives. This might be just the answer you are looking for.

ISBN 978-0-473-11228-8 (192 pages)
(NZ$34.95 Aus$34.95 US$19.95)
Available from the website: www.doctorgluten.com

Eczema! Cure It!

☐ Full of it! The Shocking Truth About Gluten

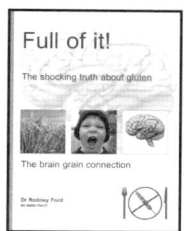

An alarming fact is that gluten can damage your brain. Have you ever wondered why you crave for another hunk of bread? If a food that you ate was slowly eroding the function and the ability of your brain, then would you want to know what that food was? It is gluten! Gluten is linked to ataxia, migraine, ADHD, autism, depression, epilepsy, mood and psychiatric disorders. Gluten also can disrupt your brain's regulation of your gut – causing mayhem in your bowel. Gluten-sensitivity is a brain disease! Read the evidence for yourself.

ISBN 978-0-473-10407-8 (192 pages)
(NZ$34.95 Aus$34.95 US$19.95)

☐ Gluten-Free Parties & Picnics

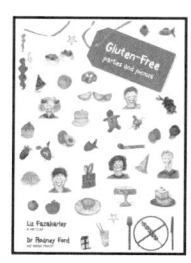

Oh dear, it's Libby's birthday – how will we manage to do a gluten-free party? How will we cope on a family picnic? These questions are answered for your children in a story-book format, in vibrant full colour. It is packed with great party and picnic ideas. Great for your family and friends to learn about the gluten-free issues. It makes it easy for your children to understand about gluten. At last an enchanting gluten book for your children.

ISBN 978-0-473-10774-1 (64 pages, full colour)
(NZ$19.95 Aus$19.95 US$14.95)

Available from the website: www.doctorgluten.com

Eczema! Cure It!   BOOK ORDER FORM

❑ **Eczema! Cure It!**

❑ ***The Gluten Syndrome***

❑ **Going Gluten-Free: How to Get Started**

❑ **Are You Gluten-Sensitive? Your Questions Answered**

❑ **The Gluten-Free Lunch Book**

❑ The book for the **Sick, Tired & Grumpy**

❑ **Full of it! The shocking truth about gluten**

❑ **Gluten-Free Parties & Picnics**

(Please indicate the number of each book that you want to order. Prices stated on previous page)
Please add postage & handling: 1 book $7.00, 2 books $12, 3 or 4 books $15
(Prices for postage and handling to be paid in the currency of purchase)

Order for:
Name: _____

Postal address: _____
_____

Phone: _____   Fax: _____

Email: _____ @ _____

Number of books required: _____   Currency _____

Cost of books $ _____   Postage $ _____   Total $ _____

Method of payment:
Cheque ❑   Visa ❑   MasterCard ❑   (please tick)

Cardholder's name: _____

Credit card number : _____

Signature: _____   Expiry date: _____ / _____

Please make your cheque payable to:
Doctor Gluten, PO Box 25-360, Christchurch, New Zealand.
Fax orders: +64 3 377 3605
Email orders: orders@doctorgluten.com
Web orders: www.doctorgluten.com
(Please allow up to 21 days for postal delivery)